Medical ethics
A CASE-BASED APPROACH

Commissioning Editor: Michael Parkinson
Project Development Manager: Fiona Conn
Project Manager: Frances Affleck
Designer: Erik Bigland

Medical ethics

A CASE-BASED APPROACH

Lisa Schwartz BA MA PhD
Chair of Health Care Ethics, McMaster University, Canada
Bioethicist, Cancer Care Ontario, Canada

Paul E Preece MB BCh MD (Wales) FRCS (Edin) FRCS (Eng) Cert THE
Senior Lecturer, Faculty of Medicine, Dentistry and Nursing, University of Dundee, UK
Formerly Consultant Surgeon, Ninewells Hospital, Dundee

Robert A Hendry MB ChB MPhil MBA MRCGP DRCOG
Adviser, Medical and Dental Defence Union of Scotland

SAUNDERS

Edinburgh • London • New York • Philadelphia • St Louis • Sydney • Toronto • 2002

SAUNDERS
An imprint of Elsevier Science Limited

First published 2002

ISBN 0 702 02543 7

British Library Cataloguing in Publication Data
A catalogue record for this book is available from the British Library

Library of Congress Cataloging in Publication Data
A catalog record for this book is available from the Library of Congress

Note
Medical knowledge is constantly changing. As new information becomes
available, changes in treatment, procedures, equipment and the use of drugs
become necessary. The authors and the publishers have taken care to ensure
that the information given in this text is accurate and up to date. However,
readers are strongly advised to confirm that the information, especially with
regard to drug usage, complies with the latest legislation and standards of
practice.

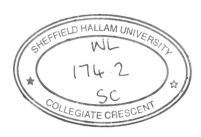

The
publisher's
policy is to use
**paper manufactured
from sustainable forests**

Printed in China

Preface

Ethical, legal and moral issues are woven seamlessly into the fabric of the practice of medicine of all types. Formal systematic study of medical ethics by students and practitioners is increasingly being recognised by medical schools, by regulatory bodies and by students as desirable, even necessary.

There are many different approaches which can be taken to doing this, ranging from the theoretical to the participatory. It is recognised that many medical students have better recall of facts they learn within the context of real cases they encounter. This book is written to deal with issues in medical ethics derived from and analysed in the context of real cases. Much of the material is universally relevant. However, contemporary debates and dilemmas have been included, together with many historic cases, the resolution of which profoundly informs current practice.

All three authors have extensive experience in teaching medical ethics to health care professionals. The viewpoint of each of us constructively compliments those of the other two. Lisa Schwartz is a professional philosopher who is senior lecturer in an academic department of general practice. Robert Hendry was a principal in a teaching general practice, until he became a medical adviser with a medical defence organisation. Paul Preece, an academic surgeon based in hospital, has co-ordinated programmes of ethics instruction for undergraduates for over 20 years. We are familiar with the needs and challenges of undergraduates, and have written the book to try to meet these for health care professionals in training.

Acknowledgements

The authors gratefully acknowledge the following:

Elsevier Science's Michael Parkinson for the initial commission, and Fiona Conn and Colin Arthur for keeping us writing and for encouraging us to create balanced comprehensive coverage.

Our students who have received and critiqued the contents of this book as teaching material over the years. We are grateful for the stimulating questions and conversations that helped clarify and guide the contents of these chapters. Also students who have allowed us to use or adapt real cases which they have encountered in their clinical attachments.

Dr Katrina Moffat, Dr Phil Cotton and Dr Margaret Greig for commenting on material.

Our respective departments for their support and time in the development of the book.

Miss Cecilia Edward, Leader of the Ethics Cognitive Group in the Schools of Nursing and Midwifery, Dundee and Kirkcaldy, whose commitment to delivering exciting and meaningful instruction to student health professionals has inspired and informed what we are attempting by writing this book.

Ms Fiona Paterson and Dr Ian G Simpson for reviewing and commenting on the chapter on Accountability.

Special thanks to Sue Brind for her invaluable guidance in finding stimulating and provocative works of art for each of the chapters. And to the artists, poet and galleries for their kind permissions and enthusiasm at being part of this book.

Special also thanks to Jane Goodfellow for her assistance with the technology and to Gillian Paton for all her help in organising meetings.

Our respective spouses, Patrick, Gill and Heather for tolerating us as we devoted more time to the book than to them.

Contents

Index of cases

I swear by the music

I swear by the music of the expanding universe
and by the eloquence of the good in all of us
that I will excite the sick and the well
by the severity of my kindness
to a wholeness of purpose. I shall apply my knowledge,
curiosity, ignorance and ability to listen.
I shall co-operate with wondering practitioners
in the arts and the sciences,
with all who care for people's bodies and souls,
so that the whole person in relationship
shall be kept in view, their aspirations and their unease.
The secrets of the universal mind
I shall try to unravel to yield beauty and truth.
The fearful and sublime secrets told to me in confidence
I shall keep safe in my heart.
I will not knowingly do harm to my patients,
I will smile at them,
and encourage them to attend to their dreams
and so hear the voices of their inner strangers.
If I keep to this oath I shall hope for the respect of my teachers,
and of my patients and of the community,
and to be healed even as I am able to heal.

David Hart
July 1987

Published with permission of the author. Originally commissioned and published by the *Observer* in July 1987.

Introduction: Why study ethics?

All individuals come with their own beliefs and values. Students of medicine and of nursing both graduate and qualify in order to practise their respective professions. As practitioners they have to subscribe to the beliefs and values of the profession of which they become part. The beliefs and values of the medical and nursing professions are deeply rooted in history. Over time, these corporate beliefs and values have been tested, even – to an extent – validated. For most individuals embarking on study of a health profession, the existing ethos of the chosen subject is itself likely to have contributed to the appeal and the vocation.

An individual wishing to become a healthcare professional has to learn the principles by which the profession works. For healthcare, these include many fundamental issues in philosophy such as humanity, personhood, relationships and society, as well as morality and regulation.

Although medicine is based on facts, i.e. it is grounded in science, the exercising of these facts requires articulate thinking, balance and judgement, which are informed by ethical considerations. Ideally, at the point of delivery, the ethics input is linked seamlessly with the scientific considerations. To achieve this level of holistic competence, medical ethics has to be taught and studied, some of this in a theoretical way. A cardiovascular analogy is that in order to be able to interpret an electrocardiogram, it is desirable to know about resting membrane potentials of cardiac muscle. In geriatrics, awareness of the concept of 'autonomy' enhances the capacity to create a care plan for a patient with Alzheimer's disease.

One of the many processes by which students of medicine become professionals is by their accepting formally the received wisdom and time-honoured principles which society considers appropriate. Assenting, either in words or in writing, to a declaration or an oath is a widely practised means of challenging the newcomer to the profession with some of these principles and values. Appendix 1 includes three examples of such oaths: the Hippocratic Oath (shown in two different versions, one old, the other contemporary), the Oath of a Muslim physician, and the Oath of Maimonides. Variations in the basic beliefs of individuals coming to the profession make it desirable, even necessary, that more than one oath should be available for the initiate to choose from, to subscribe to personally. Assenting to such a declaration is intended to bind initiates to practising these principles throughout their professional lives. In Canada, at graduation, construction engineers are given a ring to wear throughout their lives. The metal from which these rings are made comes from a bridge which collapsed, causing many deaths.[1] By way of analogy, doctors who forget the fundamental ethical principles to which they subscribe at graduation, will be liable to cause unnecessary suffering, and even death.

A further reason for formal study of medical ethics is to enhance the ability to cope with uncertainty. All human beings have to cope with uncertainty. This is especially the case for the healthcare professional, because, as such, we deal with the seeming random exigencies of biology, disease, personalities and politics. To acquire a comprehensive foundation of mainstream ethical issues relevant to health care will prepare the professional to anticipate, cope with, discuss and resolve constructively, ethical dilemmas and challenges encountered in practice every day.

In our professional lives as doctors, we will regularly encounter problems that require us to make difficult decisions. There will be times when we are not certain what the best choice of action ought to be. There will be times when our own choices, beliefs and values do not coincide with those of others. Such conflicts will arise with colleagues, other professionals, superiors, accepted guidelines and, most significantly, with patients.

Ordinarily, we tend to rely on our own intuitions and beliefs to settle these problems, but when conflicts arise it may be counterproductive to fall back on those very beliefs that are causing the conflict in the first place. Thus we require other approaches for decision making. First of all, it is natural for medical professionals to turn to medical science to help them deal with difficult problems. However, science cannot address all the problems encountered in healthcare. For example, science cannot help us decide how to break bad news to patients and their families. In fact, science cannot tell us whether family members ought to be informed at all. So, loosely we can say that science cannot provide the answers to those questions that are not quantifiable, i.e. cannot be measured in scientific terms. These are the issues that must be covered by the art of medicine.[2]

Is it enough to say that anything non-scientific that emerges in healthcare can be addressed by recourse to social values and general norms such as etiquette and good manners? Can we just leave these problems to common sense? What exactly is common sense? What is so common about it? Is common sense equipped to deal with uncommon problems? To analyse these questions, we have to consider whether:

(i) those ideas that we consider to be common sense can be agreed upon by all people at all times, or at least by most reasonable people most of the time;
(ii) common sense can supply answers to all the difficult questions faced in medicine; and
(iii) common sense is properly grounded on rational and thorough arguments that can withstand active scrutiny. The answer to these questions is very often negative. As a result, we need stronger approaches for dealing with the difficult decisions that emerge in medical care.

Some directions do exist to help guide difficult decisions. Three important approaches are:

1. laws
2. professional codes and guidelines
3. the principles and theories of ethics.

These three tools can be recruited to assist our own natural decision-making abilities, which include common sense, personal beliefs and the factual scientific knowledge we learn during the course of our undergraduate and postgraduate studies.

It is important to understand the differences between the six approaches to decision making outlined so far. To review, these are:

1. our own beliefs
2. science
3. common sense
4. laws
5. professional codes and guidelines
6. the principles and theories of ethics.

There is no clear delineation between what counts as our own beliefs and what counts as common sense. This is because, most of the time, we regard as common sense those beliefs that we have held for a long time, or which we take to be natural because they fit other beliefs we have always held. However, we can have personal beliefs that are original, or beliefs that are not compatible with the beliefs of other people. This is why we distinguish personal beliefs from common sense. Thus, personal beliefs are those that might or might not coincide with beliefs held by others, whereas common sense can be characterized by generally accepted norms.

We know that beliefs and norms are not necessarily common throughout the world. Differences in geography, socioeconomic conditions, education, history, religion and culture can produce differences in what is regarded as common sense and what is not. As a result, we have to look elsewhere to find things that can be demonstrated to be true, things that philosophers tend to call 'universal truths'. Science can help us with these to some extent but there come points where science has either not advanced enough, or where it simply isn't the right approach. Thus, science can help us to diagnose HIV anywhere in the world, but it cannot yet provide a cure for AIDS. Hopefully, in the not too distant future, science will be able to find a cure. However it will never be able to stop the prejudice that confronts some victims of HIV. To put it another way, medical science will never be able to heal prejudice. Things like prejudice involve value judgements and personal beliefs that cannot be addressed by science. Hence we look in other directions to find ways to deal with these difficult issues.

Consider law. We rely on laws to tell us how to proceed in many situations. Laws tell us: how traffic is regulated, how to keep from going to prison, how property is owned or loaned. In medicine, law can tell us how to keep records and who can write these, e.g. documents such as birth and death certificates. Law can protect patients from being taken advantage of and from being treated negligently. Law can also protect practitioners from malpractice suits, and defend them when such suits arise. The question always arises with law 'Is that which is legal, that which is right?'[3] We know that some laws are arbitrary and take the shape they do only for purposes of standardization. For example, laws about

driving vehicles on the left-hand side of British roads are convenient, but not absolute. People could get along perfectly well driving on the other side of the road, and do, where the law imposes this. Not all laws are so obviously arbitrary, though. Laws that protect us from murder do not appear arbitrary, but necessary, which is usually the case (although questions still arise about justifiable homicide, such as in self-defence, or in more opaque circumstances such as a doctor doing everything possible to end someone's suffering). Furthermore, laws can sometimes be unfair or unjust, e.g. the racist laws of the Third Reich and apartheid. Finally, laws do not or cannot address certain issues.[4] Circumstances arise where no laws exist to tell us what to do in the case at hand. A new case can direct us to the need for legislation in a certain area, but just now laws have no answer for us or are too vague to accommodate the specifics of the case. Thus we are led to conclude that laws might not always be able to guide us in making tough decisions. This conclusion is based on three limitations of laws:

1. laws can be arbitrary (even if not obviously so)
2. laws can be unjust (at least in some situations)
3. laws may not expressly address the issue at hand.

The next (and fifth) area we can turn to for help in handling difficult decisions are the regulations, codes and guidelines formulated by professional bodies. These are rules that perhaps do not apply to everybody, but which are seen to be, and are enforced as, important to the members of a professional body. The guidelines provided by the General Medical Council, and various medical associations are good examples. They are not laws, but they are reinforced with sanctions by self-regulating professions such as doctors, nurses and lawyers. These guidelines make useful reference points for handling difficult professional situations, because they have usually been carefully reasoned on the basis of general professional experience. They are enforced as standards, usually because they have been shown to be effective and true. However, they suffer from the same problems that laws suffer from – they can be arbitrary, unjust in some situations, and incomplete. Moreover, they suffer from the added difficulty that they may contradict legislation in related areas. So these codes and guidelines, although helpful and reliable, are insufficient for dealing with difficult decisions.

This leaves us with the principles and theories of ethics. Although these do not provide ready-made methods for problem solving where difficult decisions need to be made, ethics provide us with room to explore problem situations free from the restraints of rules and sanctions. Ethics permit, and in fact thrive on, disagreement, debate and conclusions that do not adhere to norms, laws or rules. Ethics do offer certain useful pointers, for example the theories of **utilitarianism** and **deontology** (or **consequentialist** and **duty-based theories**), although even these are up for debate. Philosophers are supposed to love a challenge, and any critique or alternative to the systems mentioned would be welcomed and considered. The disadvantages of ethics are fairly obvious, though: they do not provide the answers, only more suggestions. Sometimes ethicists are accused of complicating matters further, or of setting unrealistic goals for people dealing with real situations. On the whole, philosophy is better at asking questions than providing definite answers to them. Nevertheless the advantage of studying applied ethical issues from a philosophical context is the liberation it provides to anyone willing to explore and push back the limits of the expected and the accepted.

The imperfections of the previously described methods of problem solving leave us with only one option: toleration of uncertainty. As it stands today, we have no absolutes for handling difficult decisions, there are no clear signposts and there is no unequivocal way. If we did have formula answers for them, the decisions wouldn't be difficult. This means that we need to find ways of coping with the difficulties that do arise. The discussions that follow are developed to help with this.

The purpose of this discourse on the ethics of healthcare is to:

- create awareness of other perspectives
- sensitise ourselves to the reasons for our beliefs
- enable conclusions which embrace both of the above
- develop skills in constructing reasoned arguments
- introduce a variety of ethically sensitive issues in medicine.

In this text, practical cases ranging from euthanasia and abortion to informed consent and truth-telling are described. Questions will arise such as the ethical acceptability of antenatal screening for Down syndrome, and whether surrogacy is an acceptable treatment for infertility. The conflict between the rights of individuals and the best interests of the community will be contrasted with the desire of physicians to heal that rift by providing care for individual patients while at the same time being sensitive to the need to make the best use of scarce resources. Arguments will be presented to provide balanced perspectives of the positions involved. Few, if any, fixed answers will be provided as resolutions of the cases and the problems they represent. Instead, you will be provided with different views and some tools for analysing the problems, creating arguments and counter-arguments to enable you to reach your own conclusions.

Each section includes case studies to provide the backdrop for drawing out discussions about general principles and theories.[5] Different perspectives will be considered and study or discussion questions are provided. These are meant to encourage you to pursue the issues in greater depth and in conversation with colleagues and people not involved in professional healthcare delivery. The more you debate and allow your opinions to be challenged, the stronger (i.e. the more robust) these will become, and the more confident you will be as you cope with uncertainty in your professional life.

Notes and references

1. Jeswist, J. Information relevant to the Iron Ring Ceremony. http://conn.me.queensu.ca/dept/jj-ring.htm
2. Downie R., Macnaughton J. Clinical judgement: evidence in practice. Oxford: Oxford University Press, 2000.
3. Gillon, R. Imposed separation of conjoined twins – moral hubris by the English courts? Journal of Medical Ethics 2001; 27:3–4.
4. Glover S. It's time for the lawyers to stop playing God… Mail on Sunday Glasgow, 1 October 2000.
5. Pattison S., Dickenson D., Parker M. and Heller T. Do case studies mislead about the nature of reality? Journal of Medical Ethics 1999; 25: 42-46.

1

Ethical theories: some of the tools of the trade

Introduction

We don't expect the readers of this text to become experts in philosophical theory. What this book, and specifically this chapter, aims to do is offer the reader some philosophical theory that can be usefully applied to decision making in medical practice.

The following areas of philosophical enquiry will be discussed in this chapter:

- value judgements
- ethical theories.

The discussion of philosophy will be brief, in the hope that those who are interested will look elsewhere for further details on ethics and value theory. Our goal is always to retain 'that feeling for reality that ought to be preserved in even the most abstract discussions.'[1] So theories will be described here with the intention of their being applied to cases in later chapters.

How can philosophy help?

Studying philosophy can help bring the following elements to decision making in any context:

- *Clarity:* reasoned understanding of your own position
- *Plurality:* consideration and understanding of other positions
- *Awareness:* understanding criticisms of your position and preparation of counterarguments against them
- *Flexibility:* an ability to adjust your position in accordance to new events and information

- *Justification:* stated clear arguments in support of your position and decision.

It isn't enough for a doctor to hold an opinion on a matter of ethical importance distinct from, but related to, medical science. Health care professionals must also be able to justify their opinions with reasoned argument. For example, physicians might object to or support a woman's right to choose an abortion in certain cases. Either way, they could be challenged to explain their position and justify support or refusal to support the woman's choice. Reasoned justification is relevant in wider policy issues as well. For example, scientific evidence must be produced to support decisions about resource distribution, but such policies also have to be explained and justified so that those affected by the decisions understand them, and either comply with or have freedom to challenge the decisions.

If argument and justification are absent from such decisions, they will be open to weaknesses. Supported by clear and balanced arguments, a position is likely to stand strongly against even the most stringent criticisms. Nevertheless, all policies and decisions ought to be open to review for two very important reasons. First, because a position is strengthened by its ability to face up to criticism. This requires awareness of potential counterarguments and preparation for argument in response. Second, and possibly more importantly, a position must be flexible and open to change if faced with new and contradictory information and difficult unforeseen cases. Again, the ability to bend makes the position stronger, but also prevents it from succumbing to failures and oversights.

Awareness and clarity of the elements that weaken or strengthen a decision are some of the tools philosophy can provide. Examination of personal and professional opinions uncovers faulty or prejudicial reasoning that can interfere with clear understanding of a problem. This chapter describes how value judgements can interfere with and assist decision making. Later, we will describe some of the classical theories of ethics and offer potentially viable tools for assisting clarity of thought, awareness and justification in ethical decision-making. Descriptions of logical analysis are beyond the scope of this text. Those readers interested in further reading about the structure of arguments can refer to logic and critical thinking texts.[2]

Values in practice

What we value shapes the way we see the world; values shape our perspective (Fig. 1.1). Moral values are more than just attitudes; they are the foundations for judgements, decisions and actions. As people develop they accumulate preferences, likes and dislikes, knowledge and experiences that affect the way they understand and behave. Although people will have values in common, there will also be differences between values and values that are not so common. This produces disagreement. Most people form their values on the basis of experiences, education and political and religious beliefs, among other things. People trained as healthcare professionals are, through their education, given the information and experience that establish a biomedical view of the world. Philosophy of medicine reveals that the biomedical approach, like other value bases, produces a narrowing of vision that, however informative, can sometimes lead to error or clashes with the values of others. So it is important to add to this training, tools and skills for considering value differences:

> Asher was graphic in drawing attention to the dangerous tendency of clinicians to see the expected and unconsciously dismiss the anomalous: 'We have to beware of this suppressive faculty which, by producing selective deafness, selective blindness, and other sense rejections, can so easily suppress the significant and the relevant.'[3]

This is important because openness is a requirement of respectful interaction with others. If we permit our own value judgements to function without challenge, we risk imposing them on others – something doctors have been accused of doing for some time. The response has been to emphasize

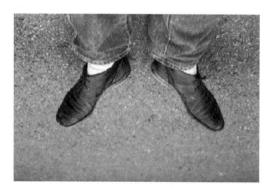 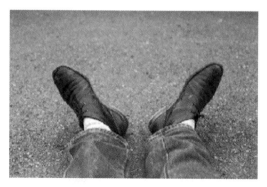

Figure 1.1
The problem with perspective is that you need to know where you stand. ('Ottawa shoes' Patrick Brennan 1989. Reproduced with kind permission of the artist.)

patient-centred approaches to care, but this risks imposing an imbalance that no one will be satisfied with. It can produce bewilderment in professionals who believed they were doing the best for their patients, but whose efforts are spurned.

Medicine involves uncertainties both as a scientific endeavour and as a human endeavour.

> Hunter, a professor of literature with a strong involvement in medical education, writes, somewhat controversially, that clinical medicine 'shares its methods of knowing with history, law, economics, anthropology and other human sciences less certain and more concerned with meaning than the physical sciences. But unlike those disciplines, it does not explicitly recognise its interpretative character or the rules it uses to negotiate meaning.' She is puzzled by the medical profession's preoccupation with the gold standard of science in clinical practice, and believes that medicine is better characterised as a 'moral knowing, a narrative, interpretative, practical reasoning.'[4]

These quotes summarize some of the criticisms made of the biomedical model of care. They show that the medical values of fact centred scientific approaches can be limiting and lead to error or oversight.

Case 1
Woman with brain tumour

Ms B, a 50-year-old registered nurse with a history of breast cancer, was brought to Accident and Emergency by ambulance. She was suffering from severe vomiting, dizziness, loss of coordination and a tingling sensation in her arms and legs. Dr R, the young attending physician, gave her a routine examination and settled on a diagnosis of flu, which was epidemic at that time. He dismissed her and told her to see her doctor if the symptoms persisted after a couple of weeks. Ms B was not satisfied with the diagnosis and was concerned that the tingling and loss of control in her limbs were signs of neurological problems. Dr R disagreed, refusing to refer Ms B for a neurological examination. Ms B persisted and, on her own efforts, made an emergency appointment with Dr G, a senior consulting neurologist in the same hospital. When Dr G heard Ms B's symptoms she was immediately certain that there was neurological involvement. After a CAT scan her diagnosis was confirmed. Ms B had a tumour inside her brain that was pushing on her cerebellum and causing the symptoms.

This case illustrates how values, and in this case biomedical conviction, shape the way we see the world. In a sense, the doctors in the case did nothing different. They each read a pattern in a set of symptoms and drew conclusions from these. Their expectations differed, however, and recognition of such differences was relevant to the application of their scientific knowledge. If the emergency care doctor had widened his expectations he might have applied the science correctly. As it was, his failure to see all the relevant symptoms led to his mistaken diagnosis. This might have been encouraged by the mitigating circumstances of the flu epidemic and his expectations could have been coloured by having seen similar symptoms caused by the flu. Lack of experience plays an appreciable role as well, but fundamentally it was worldview or value-based expectations that created the problem.

Dr G's response wasn't necessarily any different, but her world view and experience led her to have different expectations of the symptoms. Was it just luck?

Does this mean that all doctors are destined for careers of second guessing, leading to defensive tactics and futile, overcautious diagnostic procedures? Not necessarily. Instead, critics of the narrow biomedical model merely urge doctors to be open to possible change and to listen carefully to what patients tell them. In the case of Ms B, Dr R ought to have paid attention to her insistence. If he had been listening more carefully, he would probably have been more concerned by her neurological symptoms and the history of cancer.

Much (most?) uncertainty in medicine is not created by poor or impaired clinical judgement in the application of science. It is, instead, the less scientific and more humanistic factors that confound practice and lead to mistakes. The indeterminacy and relativity of values in clinical practice are what cause the uncertainty. Doctors are more frequently accused of malpractice or negligence for reasons of poor communication with patients than any other reason; hence the emphasis on developing good communication skills. The case of Ms B indicates further areas for concern. The value judgements placed on the patient by the doctors in the case are relevant to how and whether they treated her. Value judgements become an issue of significance to the less scientific human aspects of medicine as well. Assumptions are made about what is 'common sense' and what 'everyone expects'. Agreement is assumed among ethical and social values where much less agreement actually exists. Common sense is not all that common. As a result, standpoint analysts suggest that we are motivated by our worldviews and ought to at least try to be sensitive to the points of view of others – their expectations, hopes and realities – especially when the decisions directly affect their lives. Doing so involves stretches of the imagination, communication and empathy, to gain insight into the values that direct personal choice and behaviour.

Something ethical theory can help with is consideration of the ethical problems from different perspectives – at least to a point. Moral theories approach problems in different ways to highlight different values. Exploring the problems from the angles provided by different moral theories can assist decision makers to become aware of the values of others. A comparison of the results

they yield will provide insight into possible conflicts and help determine areas of agreement. This is not why the theories were developed. Each theoretical perspective has attempted to provide a realistic model for solving ethical problems, as well as for directing one in how to live a good or virtuous life. For our purposes, however, they will be used as tools. Tools for comparison and verification that consideration has been made of more than one response. Thus the tools can help us see how one ought to act if one is concerned with outcomes only, which medicine frequently is; and compare this with an alternative that is determined by concern for one's moral duty in a given situation.

A selection of accepted ethical theories will be outlined briefly in this chapter. The theories will then be employed in future chapters as tools for considering different approaches to problem solving in a variety of medical contexts and case studies.

Ethical theories

The field of ethics that studies and develops theoretical approaches to solving ethical problems is called meta-ethics. There are a number of useful and well-known approaches to ethical decision making, although none offers a flawless means of resolving ethical problems. The theories described here are selected because they are popular in applied ethics for the practical insights they yield and the values they embody.

Consequentialism[5]

This theory places moral emphasis on the consequences or outcomes of an act rather than the act itself. An action is morally correct provided its consequences are beneficial. But beneficial to whom? It might be the good of particular individuals. However, some, namely utilitarians, say it is to the greatest number of people; hence the motto: 'the greatest good for the greatest number'. When this is not possible, the action ought to cause the least amount of harm possible.

Consequentialism presents two major problems. First, it is impossible to predict beyond any doubt which act will produce the best or least harmful outcomes. As a result, consequentialism might not be capable of providing perfect help in decision making. It would require clairvoyant knowledge of actual as opposed to probable outcomes. Second, it is sometimes necessary for consequentialism to praise or blame an act for its unforeseen and unintended outcome. So, if A intends to harm B and is successful, then A is punishable according to consequentialism. But equally, if A intends to help B and instead accidentally causes B harm, then A is still punishable according to consequentialism.

Duty-based/deontology[6]

Immanuel Kant founded this theory. The emphasis here is upon the correctness of an action, regardless of the possible benefits or harm it might produce. Thus deontologists believe that there are particular duties that must be upheld at any cost. Kant's categorical imperatives are three such duties. The three formulations of the categorical imperative are:

1. Act in such a way that your actions can and ought to be universalizable
2. Treat people as ends in themselves and never solely as means to an end
3. Act in such a way as you would have others act towards you.

This theory is also concerned with the rational intentions of actors. An act is morally praiseworthy only if the actor made a reasoned choice to perform it and if the actor's intentions were morally correct. Thus accidentally correct actions are not praiseworthy; actors must intend to do their duty.

The fundamental problem with deontology is that it demands that actors perform their duty regardless of the consequences. So, for example, it would be your duty to tell the truth even though the consequences of doing so injure someone's feelings or put someone in danger. A second problem with deontology is that there is no consensus regarding a list of duties, or how to respond when two or more duties clash.

Casuistry[7]

A theory that advocates analysis of and decisions based on previous cases. This means comparing individual cases and resolutions for aspects they have in common, and basing future decisions upon these conclusions. The classic criticism of this theory points out that cases have relevant differences that could prevent them from conforming to a case type in an informative way.

Contextualism

This approach advocates making decisions on a case-to-case basis rather than using some greater theoretical framework. Contextualists believe that no two cases are identical and that treating them as such is unfair. Thus they advocate making carefully deliberated decisions within the contexts in which they arise. The chief criticism of this approach is that it is relativistic, in other words it offers no general rules or principles upon which to base judgements or make practical decisions. As a result, there is no way to predict whether or not an act will be judged to be morally acceptable.

Virtue ethics[8]

This is an Aristotelian approach based upon character and habit. It places value upon moral character rather than acts or outcomes of acts. The virtue-based approach assumes that people can act in a virtuous manner through careful training until they acquire the habit of always being virtuous. Behaving virtuously entails choosing the best approach to create happiness, or deliberating upon general principles until the best decision is reached. This theory rejects the reliance upon rules for resolving moral problems, for which it has been heavily criticized – if there are no rules to follow, how do we know we are making the virtuous decision? The response is, we know because we are virtuous. A second criticism of virtue ethics is that there is no defined set of approved virtues, so it is never certain when one is behaving virtuously and when not.

Intuitionism

This theory places attention on the role of the subject in ethical decision making. It entails understanding how we use our own moral intuitions about specific cases. Intuitionists believe that we are born with an innate ability to know right from wrong, or that we can acquire this through practice. This theory is usually considered to be an interesting beginning to ethical decision making but fails as an isolated theory because it offers no guidance beyond following a gut reaction. As a result, decisions would be based on personal prejudices instead of reasoned deliberation.

Relativism[9]

At a certain point in moral development it becomes apparent that there is scope for disagreement about what is right and what is wrong, what is acceptable and what is unacceptable behaviour, and where the locus of moral truth or certainty lies. Moral relativism is a theory that embraces this kind of difference, claiming no moral absolutes and no fixed, better way of judging right from wrong. Relativists do not argue that this is because some people are mistaken about moral truths whereas others are correct. Rather, they say that moral rules are

merely the contingent product of cultural imperatives and social customs. We judge right from wrong on the basis of what our cultural and religious customs tell us is right or wrong. As a result, we must have respect for the different attitudes of others and accept that their way could be the best way in the context of their social norms and customs. The idea of moral judgement in relativist terms occurs only within cultural contexts and must be internally consistent to be correct.

This is a useful theory in multicultural contexts where relativism makes it possible to accept and have respect for social customs that differ from one's own. In the medical context, moral relativism allows us to respect the needs of patients and practitioners with divergent customs.

The primary objection to relativism is that there is not scope for judging actions to be universally right or wrong,[10] so we could not, for example, justify statements of the sort 'torture is always wrong.'[11]

Pragmatism[12]

Ethical pragmatism is founded on philosophical exposition of American Pragmatic theorists. In essence, pragmatism is driven by the belief that there is a fundamental link between theory and practice, and that this link informs both sides. They argue that theory is a necessary guide for practice but that practice is also necessary for informing theory. Thus pragmatism makes an excellent theoretical guide for fields of applied ethics such as healthcare ethics, bioethics and business ethics. This is because it can provide direction by asserting guiding principles to ethical problems but will support the theoretical postulates with experience of how theories are realized in practice. The theory can then be modified to reflect real and practical needs and outcomes. Pragmatism uses principles for guidance but does not view these principles as immutable or infallible. Rather, pragmatists seek to understand how principles can be applied to the real world and then adjust them to ensure fit.

The obvious problem with pragmatism is that it appears overly opportunistic. It can justify almost any act or belief because the principles that provide the basis for judgement can be adjusted to accommodate almost anything. Pragmatists could even be accused of complying too readily with the winds of change and are in danger of basing moral judgements on social fashions instead of immutable truths.

Their response to this is that the need for immutable truth in ethics is founded on a mistaken belief that such things are possible or even desirable. They will reject the restrictiveness of certainty for a preferred tactic of pragmatic debate and discovery of the best way to do things for that time. They welcome empirical observation and research to inform changeable guiding principles.

Liberalism

Strictly speaking, liberalism, as outlined by John Stuart Mill, is more a political than an ethical theory.[13] Still, it does offer some relevant ethical guidelines, which are usually very popular. In its simplest form, these involve freedom and tolerance. Liberalists assert that everyone ought to be free to act as they choose provided their freedom does not interfere with similar freedom in others. Criticisms of this theory will be addressed under Ethics of care, below.

Ethics of Care

Feminist scholars such as Carol Gilligan developed this theory.[14] It is a direct response to the inherent coldness of liberal tolerance, which proponents of the Ethics of Care saw as leaving some people out in the cold. 'Caring' advocates decision making in a way that best supports the good of the individual in the long run. An Ethic of Care requires us to assume responsibility for those who need

our help, and to do whatever it takes to further their best interests. Care involves compromise in order to work out the best possible solution, even if this means changing the rules. Hence, sometimes we will interfere with the autonomous actions of others in order to preserve or enhance their future autonomy. Ethics of Care is usually criticized as a disguise for paternalism. Critics describe this theory as interfering for the good of patients even when patients are able to make their own decisions and do not seek the interference.

Rights

A right is a means of protecting a form of behaviour that is considered valuable in its own right. Thus, a right could be considered to be a special form of behaviour that needs no justification. Rights always need some kind of assistance to be upheld. For example, a person could have a right to medical care but cannot fulfil this right without hospitals, medicines and professional caregivers. It follows from this that rights confer duties. A right confers a duty when someone must help the right-holder to accomplish a desire or fulfil a need. There are two types of rights, and these are distinguished by the sort of duties they confer:

1. *Positive rights:* require others to actively support them. For instance, education and healthcare require others actively to assist right-holders to accomplish their ends. Positive rights confer active duties.
2. *Negative rights:* require non-interference on the part of others. For example, a person could have a right to walk down the street unmolested. This confers a duty upon others not to waylay the right-holder. Negative rights usually hold greater weight than positive rights. Negative rights confer passive duties.

Sanctions ensure rights are properly supported by their required duties. Thus, one can be punished if one does not perform the required positive duty associated with a positive right, or when one interferes with the negative right of another.

There is a possibility of competing rights. This occurs when more than one right is at stake and both cannot be upheld simultaneously; or when the rights of two or more individuals conflict. The conflict can arise between individuals, between individuals and communities, between communities, and even within the set of rights held by a single individual. The result of the conflict is an ethical problem.[15]

Principlism

Beauchamp and Childress first outlined this contemporary theory of applied ethics in 1983.[16] Their claim is that a decision is ethically sound provided certain principles are respected and balanced. They proposed four principles, although proponents have since suggested other candidates. Unfortunately, this indicates a failing in the theory, as no definite set of principles has been defined. Moreover, even among the principles that are agreed upon, there is no hierarchy to resolve conflicts between competing principles. Nevertheless, this has become one of the most popular theories in healthcare ethics and the principles provide helpful insights into ethical problem solving. The most commonly applied principles are listed below.

Autonomy

The ability of a person to be self-determining and self-governing;[17] the capacity of a person to make reasoned choices on the basis of information. It implies a duty on the part of caregivers to do what is necessary to promote, or at least not hinder, their patients' autonomy. This requires respect for persons, by not interfering with their plans, ambitions and choices (recall Kant's categorical imperative regarding ends and means). Autonomy is the primary consideration in patient-centred treatment.

Beneficence/non-maleficence

These are related concepts. Beneficence requires the caregiver to do good and help people; non-maleficence is the Hippocratic requirement on the caregiver to do no harm. If only beneficence was required of a medical practitioner, it would be impossible to maintain because it entails no limits. Thus the requirement is balanced, so at the very least the caregiver ought to do no harm. However, even this principle is not satisfactory on its own, as practitioners do occasionally have to cause some harm, such as the sting of a needle or a noxious treatment like chemotherapy. Thus we rely on beneficence to ensure that the harm is performed for a greater end.

Justice

This is an elusive concept. In some of the literature it means to treat people fairly. This might entail treating equals equally wherever possible. However, it might also mean treating some people differently when their differences are relevant. So we might choose to provide more healthcare to low-income areas where health problems are often greater and healthcare is traditionally less accessible. Some philosophers believe justice means equality of distribution of resources, while others claim it requires only equality of access.

Utility

Make the best use of resources.[18] This is to remind caregivers that they have a responsibility to the entire community, and therefore the needs of one must be carefully balanced with the needs of the many. Utility is one of the governing principles in rationing and distribution of resources (see Chapter 9).

Truth

Always be truthful in dealings with people. This helps preserve the trust that is so essential in the doctor–patient relationship. Patients need to be able to rely on the truth of what they are told if they are to make rational decisions and act autonomously.

Paternalism

Although not an ethical theory, paternalism is a term so frequently used in the context of medical ethics that it ought to be given some special analysis here. Paternalism can be described as:

> Making a decision on behalf of someone else or pre-empting a decision that they are able to make on their own behalf, on the grounds that it is for their own good.

Paternalism is common in healthcare settings where caregivers are torn between their feelings of duty to be beneficent and their desire to respect the autonomy of their patients. The human duality of autonomy and need makes it necessary to consult authorities. Authorities might know best what skills and information to apply but they lack the relevant information about the individual. Only individuals can know this with any certainty; only they are authorities about themselves. Hence, the authorities have limited expertise in particular cases because their expertise cannot include the patients' knowledge of themselves.

Because decisions are influenced by personal and professional values, decisions made by carers will often not be those the patients would have made. This is because their value bases are different and not because the patients are incompetent. Competence is related to paternalism because incompetent patients might require decisions to be made for them. Who ought to make these decisions? Does an advance directive make a difference? Do patients' past values have any bearing in decision-making for currently incompetent patients? These questions will be explored throughout the text.

Ethics of Care illustrates that there might be a degree to which paternalism is justifiable. Those who support this view assert that we are losing clinical freedom and opportunities to be beneficent if we reject paternalism altogether. In response, antipaternalists remind us that active involvement can help relieve patients' fears and help them regain control of their lives. Partnership is therefore frequently suggested as an alternative to paternalism. So what do we do with bizarre choices some patients might make? Give them 'equal footing with other choices unless some defect in the process by which they were reached can be specified'.[19]

These are just brief descriptions of some of the ethical theories that can be applied to the medical context. They have been chosen for their frequency of use in medical ethics literature. It is clear, and perhaps frustrating, that no one theory is best and that each has disadvantages. This does not mean that they are of no use. As explained above, their usefulness will be as tools for discovery and comparison. When attempting to resolve ethical conflict, the theories can be used to help uncover different points of view, different values and different ways of proceeding. So, in the context of the case of Ms B (see p. 3), one can ask 'How would a deontologist regard the doctor's actions?' or 'How would a consequentialist judge the outcome?' and thereby consider whether the caregivers discharged their duties appropriately or which of them produced the best outcome.

Many of the theories and issues discussed here will resurface in greater detail in future chapters. All of them will be useful for case study analysis in this text and we hope you will find them useful in your work as well. We have tried to formulate their use in a decision-making tool that can be applied to any case. This tool is not intended to act as a decision-making algorithm to produce perfect results. Rather, it is merely a suggestion of a means of proceeding that includes many of the relevant factors discussed in the book. It is one of many possible models and is not intended to be definitive. We hope you will use it to assist in clarifying and justifying your decisions.

Ethical decision-making tool[20]

1. Getting the story straight

Gather the relevant information and describe it as succinctly as possible. Identify stakeholders' values, as well as clinical and social issues.

2. Your initial reaction

State and consider your 'gut reaction' to the case. This helps clarify your own position before moving on to consider other people's position. You might not change your opinion, but you should be open to the possibility.

3. Identify the ethical problem(s)

Consider the difference between ethical and medical issues.

4. Duties and outcomes

What are the caregivers' duties and what outcomes ought to be produced?
Do these conflict? Which should be given priority?

Duties:

Outcomes:

5. Alternative courses of action

What alternatives are open to the healthcare provider(s)? Consider the possible risks and benefits to the patient.

Alternative 1

Alternative 2

Alternative 3

6. Principles

Consider the relevance of the following ethical principles to the alternative courses of action (N/A = not applicable):

	Alternative 1 Supports Y N N/A	Alternative 2 Supports Y N N/A	Alternative 3 Supports Y N N/A
Patient autonomy (self-governance and self-determination):			
• Truth			
• consent			
• confidentiality			
Beneficence (promote good):			
Non-maleficence (do no harm):			
Justice (equitable distribution of benefits and burdens in society):			
Utility (make best use of overall resources):			

7. Legal and professional requirements

What are the relevant laws and professional requirements?

8. Reflection on the answers so far

9. Decision

Make and articulate a resolution for this case [this might be (i) a clear preference; (ii) an uncertain preference, (iii) no preference].

10. Justify your decision

This is very important. All decisions must be fully explained and supported.

11. Anticipate criticisms and costs

What will the critics say about your position? How will you respond?

12. Implement and document

Put the decision into action and keep a progress record.

13. Reflection and evaluation

Consider the effects and impact of your decision for the patient, the caregivers, the medical context and society in general.

14. Reconsideration

Be open to the possible need to reconsider and change your decision.

Exercise
Before proceeding any further, it will be useful to take a moment to reflect on your own beliefs and ideas about medical practice. Ask yourself 'What are the ideals of medical practice?' and 'What should a good doctor be good at?' Write your responses in the space provided. Then consider what would be the minimal requirements for adequacy. Keep a note of your thoughts handy. You will find it helpful to refer to the list in consideration of the various cases and challenges raised in future chapters.[21]

What are the ideals of medical practice?

What is the good doctor good at?

Notes and references

1 Russell B. Introduction to Mathematical Philosophy, p. 169. London: Allen & Unwin; 1919.
2 Walton DN. Informal logic: a handbook for critical argumentation. Cambridge, MA: Cambridge University Press; 1989.
3 Greenhalgh T, Hurwitz B. Narrative based medicine: why study narrative? Br Med J 1999; 318:48–50.
4 Greenhalgh T, Hurwitz B. Narrative based medicine: why study narrative? Br Med J 1999 318:48–50.
5 Internet Encyclopaedia of Philosophy: http://www.utm.edu/research/iep/c/conseque.htm
6 Kant E. Groundwork for a metaphysics of morals, 1785
7 Jonsen AR, Toulmin S. The abuse of casuistry: a history of moral reasoning. Berkeley, CA: University of Berkeley Press; 1988.
8 London AJ. Amenable to reason: Aristotle's rhetoric and the moral psychology of practical ethics. Kennedy Institute of Ethics Journal 2000; 10 (December):4.
9 See: The Internet Encyclopaedia of Philosophy. Available: http://www.utm.edu/research/iep/m/m-relati.htm and Bernstein R. Beyond objectivism and relativism. Philadelphia: University of Pennsylvania Press; 1983.
10 Macklin R. Against relativism: cultural diversity and the search for ethical universals in medicine. New York: Oxford University Press; 1999.
11 Rachels J. The Elements of Moral Philosophy 3rd edition. McGraw Hill, 2000.
12 See: LaFollette H. Blackwell guide to ethical theory. Oxford: Blackwell; 2000. Available: http://www.etsu-tn.edu/philos/faculty/hugh/pragmati.htm and Peirce CS. Writings of Charles S. Peirce: a chronological edition, vol. 3. Bloomington, IN: Indiana University Press; 1986:242–338 and Parker K. Public hearings/hearing publics: a pragmatic approach to applying ethics. Available: http://www2.gvsu.edu/~parkerk/kp/publhear.html
13 Mill JS. On liberty. Indianapolis: Bobbs-Merrill, 1956.
14 Gilligan C. In a different voice. Cambridge, MA: Harvard University Press; 1982.
15 Dworkin R. Taking rights seriously. London: Duckworth; 1978.
16 Beauchamp TL, Childress JF. Principles of Biomedical Ethics. Oxford: Oxford University Press; 1983.
17 Downie R, Calman K. Healthy respect. Oxford: Oxford University Press; 1994.
18 Downie R, Calman K. Healthy respect. Oxford: Oxford University Press; 1994.
19 Brown J et al. Challenges in caring: explorations in nursing and ethics. London: Chapman and Hall; 1992:65.
20 This decision model was devised from many other similar tools, including the McMaster Model developed by the Faculty of Health Sciences Ethics Education Committee, McMaster University, 1993.
21 This exercise was developed for the Core Values in Medicine Exercise designed by Ken Kipnis and Anita Gerhard at the University of Hawaii School of Medicine.

2

Clinical relationships

This chapter acts as an overview of the many ethically charged issues examined in the rest of the book. We will introduce notions of professional behaviour and expectations, explore challenges to decision making and accountability in team approaches to care, and discuss the needs of especially vulnerable patients. Throughout, the duties and expectations placed on doctors will be discussed and sometimes questioned to help clarify their basis. In the final section, the impact of genetics on healthcare will be used to illustrate the many difficulties facing members of the healthcare professions and the patients they seek to help.

The details

From the moment of the first meeting between the doctor and the patient, the encounter has an ethical as well as an interpersonal and professional dimension. As with all professional encounters, be it lawyer with client or actor with audience, preparation is required. Appearance, attitude, dress, hygiene (including oral as well as axillary) and punctuality are aspects that new medical students, as well as established practitioners, need to consider. You cannot help whether you have acne or are bald, but you can help having halitosis or being late. Thinking of your appearance and your punctuality are actions that signify, non-verbally, to your patients and colleagues the fact that you respect them. Such expressions of respect can be enhanced by standing up when your patient enters the consulting room and, if culturally acceptable, shaking the patient's hand. These little gestures build confidence within the patient, which could pay dividends later in the relationship. Although in a

nationalized health service the issue of the patient paying the doctor for medical services rarely arises, consideration of this component in the relationship can generate an element of humility and subservience, which could counter tendencies towards the arrogant paternalistic veneer with which medical practitioners are so often stereotyped.

However, an attitude of openness to patients should be prevented from becoming overfriendly or familiar. The relationship is professional, not social. Although many normal social mores apply, many are suspended in the doctor–patient relationship and the manner of the doctor may need to convey this.

Communication skills

Communication skills are fundamental to good doctor–patient relationships. The task of developing these skills, together with developing awareness of the significance of body language and non-verbal communication, is integral to an ethical approach, in obtaining implicit and explicit consent, and so informing patients about what they are consenting to. In extreme situations, achieving good communications could necessitate the use of a translator.

In the case below, the confidentiality aspect had to be sacrificed in favour of achieving adequate communication. This case illustrates how vital and how enhancing to the quality of a consultation a translator can be. Signing for deaf people, as well as information and consent sheets in Braille for visually impaired people are other means by which quality can be achieved in communication, essential for the needs of the patient.

Case 2
Patient respect

A 28-year-old man from Bangladesh presented to the Casualty department with abdominal pain that had been present for 2 days. A letter from the GP accompanied the patient, but this contained only his name, date of birth and the fact that he had acute abdominal pain.

The patient was unaccompanied and could neither speak nor understand English. Although the hospital had its own Bangladeshi translator, this person was not available at this time. Being unable to take a history, let alone elicit reliably the physical signs, the house-officer asked the people in the Casualty waiting room if anybody could speak the patient's language. A man who was accompanying his own relative could speak both languages and agreed to act as interpreter. With the help of the translator, the house-officer took the patient's medical history. When it was time to examine the patient, the translator waited outside the curtain screen while the house-officer called out instructions and the translator in turn relayed these to the patient.

Working in teams and with other professionals

Chapter 4 describes in detail many aspects of 'accountability'. To show empathy is part of being accountable and empathy is usually expected and required from an individual. The quality (or attitude) of empathy is the skill of demonstrating to the client or patient that the professional is imagining vividly what it is like to be in the position of the individual who is suffering. Teamworking, especially when this is concerned with caring for and managing patients, also carries with it the expectation – indeed the requirement – that it be 'accountable'. On the one hand, shared responsbility should be less burdensome than individual responsibility; on the other hand, teamworking can make accountability more burdensome and difficult to identify and deliver. For example, it is more difficult for a patient to be empathized with by a team rather than by an individual. However, it is possible to do it.

In what ways do you think working in a team would make accountability:

1. Easier to achieve?

2. More difficult to achieve?

We will now think about multiprofessional teams in healthcare. In its instructions to practitioners and medical students, the General Medical Council emphasizes the benefits that ensue for patients when their healthcare is delivered by a team.[1] Recognition of teamworking and training for this are now a requirement in British medical schools.[2] Teamworking and delivery of healthcare by teams have potential advantages and disadvantages for both patients and professionals.[3]

Advantages for patients

- Access to greater knowledge and skills
- Benefit of a 'second opinion'
- Larger pool of resources from which patient needs can be met, e.g. beds, personnel, drug tariffs
- Opportunity for clearer information and greater emotional and psychological support
- Caregivers are involved in monitoring of practice, peer review, mutual quality assurance.

Disadvantages for patients

- Antipathy between colleagues who have different approaches, backgrounds and styles
- Time taken to reach decisions about management, i.e. consensus is prolonged (compared with a decision being made by individual practitioners on their own)
- Perceived reduction in leadership status – diluting the apparent locus of 'authority' of a single-handed practitioner
- Conflicting or divergent opinions about management
- Confusion about 'what is best'
- Possibility of 'falling between two stools'
- Delay/loss of case records and results between team members.

Similarly, advantages and disadvantages exist for the doctor as well.

Advantages for doctors

- Access to specialized advice and treatment outwith their own specialities
- Shared care and responsibility; i.e. when a patient deteriorates, as happens to patients with advanced malignancy, it is easier for a doctor to cope when sharing the management with a colleague
- Shared follow-up opportunities, resulting in less pressure on one particular facility, such as an outpatient clinic
- Broader horizons arising from multidisciplinary teams results in increased job satisfaction
- Support to help avoid mistakes and account for them afterwards if they occur.

Disadvantages for doctors

- Takes time to communicate and have case conferences
- Takes patience to counter the 'devil's advocacy' that is an integral part of case conferences
- The feeling of lack of autonomy – knowing that decisions made by oneself will be subject to discussion by colleagues from another speciality
- Comments and guidance given can be interpreted as criticism
- 'Prima donna' doctors can feel a loss of authority.

In 'real-life', individuals becoming patients cannot choose which professionals make up the team that looks after them. Recognition by the professionals that they are part of a team is, in itself, a positive feature for their patients. Information about the structure of the team, and the identity, roles and status of the professionals who form the team, is desirable, even invaluable, for the patient. Possessing this knowledge makes patients better equipped to comply with the requests made by individual team members. It also ensures that the conditions necessary for efficient team functioning are met. Ideally, all professionals in the team will function as advocates for the patient. In practice, one professional often majors in this role and efficiency is achieved by others letting this happen.

There are desirable, even proven, qualities that facilitate multiprofessional working both in healthcare and in other walks of life. Experience indicates that one of these is that the role and status of each contributing professional should be clearly conceptualized. However, it is necessary that this perception is held with flexibility, even liberality, in interpretation and implementation of these roles. Clear knowledge of where the ultimate responsibility lies for particular actions is another important component. Clearly, this assists in the precise designation of who is accountable for what. Carefully, even persistently, fostered respect for individuals of professions other than one's own is a third feature that catalyses efficient teamworking.

In theory, the functioning of a team of professionals can be enhanced by psychometric methods. These generate an inventory of the strengths inherent in the individuals who make up that team.[4] In itself, the willingness of individuals to cooperate by completing the necessary ratings scales and pooling rather personal facts about themselves can contribute to positive group (team) dynamics. The insights – of oneself and one's colleagues – obtained when completing the ratings scales could enhance productive interaction and the acquisition of insight and knowledge about oneself as a person in a working relationship with others seems to be beneficial. Overall, the use of the Belbin rating scheme seems to be withstanding the test of time (although this view is not held unanimously).

Finally, in applying the word 'team' to the complex organizational interaction within a healthcare setting, it is helpful to reflect on the following significant point. Whereas, ideally, there is a clearly identified goal for which all individuals should be working in the best interests of the patient, in practice the common goal for a healthcare team is much less clear than that of, for example, a sports team. In the healthcare setting there are frequently conflicts of interest within the coalition. Further, there are differences between the dynamics of the coalition and also differences in the extent of the commitment to the patient. Table 2.1 shows qualities that contribute to successful health teamwork and Table 2.2 lists the characteristics that are inimical to successful teamwork.[5]

Table 2.1
Qualities contributing to successful teamwork[5]

- Dedicated time and place to meet
- Tolerance of self-examination
- Understanding of group dynamics
- Stability and consistency in group members

Table 2.2
Characteristics resulting in unsuccessful teamwork[5]

- Hierarchy
- Insistence on priority of own discipline
- Reluctance to participate in team meetings
- Stereotyped attitude
- Confusion of opinions with facts

Advocacy[6]

The case of the man from Bangladesh (see p. 20) illustrates how people are rarely more vulnerable than when they are ill. As a result of this vulnerability, patients can sometimes find themselves needing someone to act on their behalf to ensure their best interests are respected. In such cases an advocate might be designated to assist the patient, although more often than not someone self-designates on the patient's behalf. We will consider the concept of the patient advocate and the challenges it involves. This will include an examination of the inherent tensions in advocacy and an attempt to answer the questions 'Who needs an advocate', 'What is an advocate?', 'Who should be the advocate?'.

An advocate can be described as one who:

- represents the values, interests and desires of another
- speaks for, or on behalf of, another.

There are strong reasons for rejecting the notion that patients need advocates at all. Healthcare professionals are trained to look out for the best interests of patients, and duties of care such as beneficence and nonmaleficence reinforce this.[7] However, differences of opinion do arise among healthcare providers and between professionals and patients. In some cases, overzealous practitioners who believe they know best have overridden patient autonomy. As a result, all patients are likely to need an advocate at one time or another, but some patients are obviously more in need of having their needs represented than others. Unconscious patients, incompetent patients, confused and frightened patients are all candidates for advocacy because of their vulnerability. The advocate's role should be to:

- protect the rights and interests of patients where they cannot protect their own[8]
- inform the patient in aid of consent
- empower the patient and protect autonomy

- ensure patients receive their fair share of resources[9]
- support the patient no matter what the choice or cost
- represent the views and/or desires of patient[5], and not just their needs.

However, the list reveals two tensions inherent in advocacy. First, there is a tension between what can be expected as an essential duty of the healthcare professional and what might legitimately be said to go beyond the expectations of care. Is advocacy an aspect of all professional healthcare? Arguably, it presents specific challenges that most people are not trained to perform and, in specific circumstances, certain dangers for healthcare professionals. These will be discussed below.

Second, there is a fine line between representation and paternalism in advocacy. It is unclear if a patient advocate is one who will represent patient values or one who will decide on behalf of the patient's best interests.

Who should be the patient's advocate?

Patients representing themselves benefit from enhanced autonomy and informed consent. But patients are in varying states of vulnerability and might be unable to represent themselves adequately. Therefore external support is beneficial if not necessary.

Family and friends as advocates
Family and friends can know a patient's needs and wishes well and, generally speaking, have an emotional investment in ensuring the best for the patient. This makes them informed and deeply committed. But the commitment can be high in demands on time and energy; it could require sacrifice in other areas of their lives, as well as struggles to be taken seriously by healthcare professionals who do not recognize them as equals in the decision-making process (and who might also be vying for the role of advocate). Also, family and friends might have vested interests in manipulating or misrepresenting the patient,

as the outcome usually affects them as well. Thus, there is a danger of covert paternalism – or worse, self-service – when family and friends act as patient advocates.[10]

Professional advocates
Experiments in professional advocacy have taken place in Austria[11] and Canada. The advocates were employed to do nothing other than advocate for the patient – they had no other loyalties and no conflicts of interest. Professional advocates can be trained and could even have some professional medical background. Their official status would reduce intimidation by the healthcare setting and protect them from being ignored.

But the very nature of a professional advocate creates an adversarial atmosphere between patient and carers that might not be natural and that could hinder patient care. Also, professional advocates are strangers to the patient and therefore might be incapable of accurately assessing patient values and goals. These are fundamental flaws in professional advocacy.

Doctors as advocates
Doctors have often claimed the role of patient advocate and there are sound justifications to support this. It could be seen as a very natural part of their jobs, as they do it all the time in the form of treatment decisions. Where GPs are concerned, there are even greater reasons to believe they will make good advocates. They often have long-standing relationships with patients and therefore have a sound basis for knowledge of a patient's goals and needs. However, recent transformation to fundholding and cooperatives in the UK, and managed care in the US, creates conflicts of loyalties between duty to patients and duty to the community.[12] Because of this, doctors might be unable to commit fully to advocating for a single patient. Also, they have historically been accused of covert paternalism and thus are not trusted to respect patient interests as the

patient perceives them. Giving doctors official status as advocates could increase their justification to act paternalistically and worsen the situation. Finally, the special difficulties that confront nurse advocates also apply to doctors, and might result in them compromising themselves in the role of advocate. These are considered in greater detail in the next section, Nurses as advocates.

Nurses as advocates

The literature contains convincing arguments in favour of nurses assuming the role of patient advocate.[13] Nurses are medically educated, professional members of the team. They tend to spend the most time with hospitalized patients and are therefore more able to assess their needs and aspirations (beyond medical needs). Moreover, the United Kingdom Central Council of Nursing (UKCC) indirectly endorses the role.[14,15] But is this right?

First, nurses, like doctors, could have conflicts of interest, as expressed in the UKCC document.[15] The interests of society and duties to the professions might conflict with adequate representation of the patient, such as when a patient requests expensive, experimental or clinically less preferred forms of treatment.[16]

Second, advocacy implies being prepared to be adversarial, and this can promote discord with colleagues and in teams.[17] Doctors face the same problem, but it can be especially -challenging for nurses, who are traditionally seen as owing their full loyalties to the doctor. Shifting the locus of loyalty towards the patient can cause disharmony and disappointment from those who expect the traditional role. This might change over time, but potential conflict with colleagues over patient wishes will be an ongoing problem.

Third, the advocate might be asked to represent a patient's bizarre or dangerous choices, or to represent a patient in ways that compromise the advocate's personal or professional beliefs. The advocate might withdraw from this, but that forces us to question whether, in doing so, they continue to be patient representatives or if their withdrawal is paternalistic. Perhaps it will be necessary to regulate the decision to quit being a patient's advocate to protect both patients and the person acting as advocate.[18]

Finally, at present there is no formal training for nurses or doctors to represent patients in this way.[19] It is true that the elements of nursing and medical education are useful for these purposes, but people who assume the role of advocate ought to be prepared for coping with the potential hazards and hardships that accompany advocacy. Knowledge of medical law and ethics will surely be useful,[20] but other qualities, such as negotiation skills and communication skills, are not as easily acquired.

Summary

It could be said that advocates would not be needed if all healthcare professionals did their jobs properly.[21] If they are going to be used, their role must be made clearer.[22] Most significantly, we need to determine whether advocacy means supporting any decision a patient makes, even bizarre or bad ones. Protection and support for advocates is needed, especially if compromise of personal or professional beliefs is required to fulfil the role adequately. For example, advocacy might require the professional to breach confidentiality[23] or to take on the responsibility of blowing the whistle on their colleagues, with all the professional discord that would result.

Anyone assuming the role of advocate will need to be prepared to deal with these compromises and also, very importantly, to be aware enough of their actions to guard against overriding patient autonomy.

Certain patients will always need some form of guidance and advocacy. We now turn to consider patients who are especially vulnerable.

Special cases in the clinical relationship

- Children (minors)
- Subjects with mental disorders and disabilities.

Children

Special considerations in the clinical relationship exist when the patient is particularly vulnerable. It is accepted that being a patient at all puts the individual into a position that has some degree of vulnerability about it. Where the patient is a child, special vulnerability exists by virtue of years, stature, immaturity, inexperience and dependency on others. This very vulnerability requires of the doctor the necessity to exercise increased responsibility. This is delivered by gentleness and patience in communicating with and examining a child, and by delicate handling of small soft tissues and viscera. In the UK, individuals aged under 18 years are legally 'minors', i.e. subject to authority of and control by their parents or guardians. However young people over the age of 16 are presumed to have the competence to give or withold their consent to investigations or treatment. Indeed children under the age of 16 can also give their consent if they have the ability to understand what is involved.[24,25,26] As a consequence, doctors - managing children deal with two clients, both of whom require consideration, communication and recognition of, and respect for, their rights.[27]

In practice, during development from birth to adulthood, there is an 'evolution' of maturity, responsibility and self-awareness in minors. This varies between individuals and, like physical growth, does not increase smoothly but occurs in alternating slow and fast phases. When children and young people have to receive medical care, they frequently show comprehension and cooperation with what their doctors and nurses ask of them, which enables the professional to establish a positive and meaningful relationship. In this circumstance, it is important for the doctor to remember that the patient is a vulnerable child, so that all measures are taken to ensure minimum pain and the least separation from the family.

Although in the majority of cases, child, doctor and parent will all agree on medical management, the necessity for three-sided agreement does produce, from time to time, disagreements and ethical and legal problems. Broadly these can be thought of in three categories:

1. Where the parent disagrees with the management the doctor is convinced the child needs
2. Where the child (minor) requests medical treatment with which the doctor will acquiesce but to which the parent(s) are opposed
3. Where the parent and the doctor wish an intervention that the child does not want.

Examples of the first category are reported regularly in the media. The scenario that has acquired classic status is that of the child of a Jehovah's Witness, who has a haemorrhage of such proportions that, unless blood is transfused, the child will die. In a number of such cases, the child has been made a ward of court, by a legal process that temporarily transfers the rights of the parents to consent for their child, to a court of law. Clearly, this measure is justified only because it is seen as the only way to save the life of the minor. It is highly damaging to the doctor–parent relationship and, in view of the beliefs of Jehovah's Witnesses about the consequences of blood transfusion, it could result in serious damage to the parent–child relationship. (We will not describe in detail what Jehovah's Witnesses believe about blood transfusion; note 28 provides a full explanation.) Another common example of this category, but where the parental disapproval does not necessarily arise from a religious belief, is when a parent declines to allow a child to be immunized against a prevalent life-threatening infectious disease. Whereas in this circumstance the death of the child is less obviously imminent, such that many doctors will reluctantly accept parental refusal, there are a number of such children who have been immunized as wards of court.

Examples from the second category also receive media attention. The most recent noteworthy example went to court and, as a result, had a significant influence on current legislation. The Gillick case is a historic landmark in British medical ethics and law. (Gillick V. West Norfolk and Wisbech AHA [1985] 3 ALL ER 402). It has given its name to a principle that informs the relationship between doctors, minors and parents. The case came about when Mrs Victoria Gillick, who has four daughters who at the time (1982) were aged under 16 years, decided to challenge in the courts Department of Health and Social Services advice given to doctors in a circular of 1974, and revised in 1980. This advice was designed to reduce the number of pregnancies and abortions in girls under 16 years of age. Broadly, the circulars permitted doctors to prescribe oral contraceptives to such minors, even in the absence of parental consent or knowledge, provided the child was considered mature enough to understand the consequences of treatment.

The case was protracted. Having been heard once in an ordinary court, it went on to the Court of Appeal and subsequently to the House of Lords. From this the Gillick principle emerged. This principle recognizes the evolving maturity of children. It empowers doctors to make an assessment of the sufficiency of the maturity that individual children have reached, so, in practice, doctors can decide in each case whether the child in front of them at the time can give valid consent for the particular medical intervention requested or required. Clearly this principle is the opposite one from that which Mrs Gillick was seeking. For doctors, although it gives a considerable measure of freedom in dealing with minors, it also invests them with onerous responsibilities in determining the maturity possessed by individual children. In practice,

when a doctor decides that a minor who is seeking a medical intervention without parental consent or knowledge is 'Gillick competent' it is vital that the characteristics observed by the doctor in the child, which resulted in this decision, are carefully and clearly recorded in the case notes.

Examples of the third category are less publicized, although must frequently be encountered. It is easy to imagine situations in which parents and doctors consider a medical intervention or a medical procedure desirable, or even life saving, but the youngster does not want it. The ethical issues always have to be judged on the merits of the individual case, e.g. is it right to perform tonsillectomy on a small child who has suffered recurrent sore throats? If, however, the child is deemed to be competent and refuses treatment, over-riding that decision is a very serious step. The ethical quandary might be resolved by finding the evidence from follow-up reviews, or even from clinical trials.

Subjects with mental disorders and disabilities

Adults are always assumed to be competent unless demonstrated otherwise. Individuals with mental disorders are especially vulnerable in a host of ways. An initial classification of these conditions usefully distinguishes permanent from temporary mental incapacity.

An example of permanent mental incapacity is an individual with retarded intellectual and personality development, such as a person who, whilst continuing to mature physically at the appropriate rate, fails emotionally and intellectually to continue to mature. Although such individuals look like 'normal' adults, their mental age is frequently well within that reckoned by our society and law as being in the bracket of 'minor'. Such individuals are clearly very vulnerable to being misled, misinformed and taken advantage of. Because of this, it is appropriate that doctors treat such individuals in a highly respectful, sensitive and careful manner, particularly in obtaining consent for medical interventions.

There are very many examples of temporary mental incapacity. In fact, it is probable that, at some time in our lives, most of us will pass through a phase of temporary mental incapacity. Doctors should keep this fact constantly in mind, because many physical, psychological and social factors can cause temporary mental incapacity. The challenge for doctors is to recognize when conditions like confusional states or depression have set in. There are well-described physical signs by which doctors can suspect these abnormalities. A further challenge arises from the fact that temporary mental incapacity can fluctuate. That is to say that patients can slip in and out of temporary mental incapacity, sometimes with disarming speed. The fact that people with temporary mental incapacity are particularly vulnerable is fundamentally important. Where it is established, or suspected, the caring, prudent doctor will focus firmly in the welfare of the patient, and take special care to ensure that, when information is given and consent requested, these activities are witnessed and what is said and done is written down. No one can give consent on behalf of an incompetent adult except in Scotland where recent legislation provides for some people to be given appropriate authority to do so. Such patients may be treated, however, if it is in their best interersts. When deciding what is in a patient's best interests account must be taken of any views they previoulsy expressed, including an advance directive, the family's and carers' knowledge of the patient's background and which options for treatment least restrict future choices.[29]

The impact of genetics on clinical relationships

Among the most ethically charged developments in medical science of the past century is the possibility of understanding and inter- vening at such a basic and minute level as our genetic make-up. The programme, the elements, the essence of 'who we are' physically, is being understood and examined thoroughly and in detail. This includes information more personal and individual than a fingerprint. A London artist, Pam Skelton, recently produced a series of paintings that she described as portraits of her friends. The exhibition catalogue, called *Pamela Hurwitz and her friends*,[30] illustrates several large canvases on which are painted the DNA of each of the models along with a smaller image of their faces. There is no doubt that this is a version of portraiture that could only have been made in the very last years of the twentieth century. Will we soon reach a point where people can be readily identifiable by the image of their DNA? If it does become possible to identify the individual with a certain genetic structure, then how might that impact on the notion of ownership and appropriation of these genes?

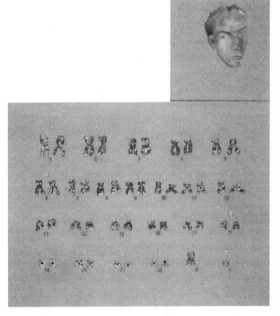

Figure 2.1
Pamela Hurwitz and her friends © Pam Skelton). A version of portraiture that could only have been made in the late twentieth century.

Issues related to genetics and reproduction are addressed in Chapter 8, including considerations about cloning and antenatal screening. In *this* section we will consider the impact of genetic information and manipulation on disease and treatment, paying particular attention to privacy and ownership of genetic information. We will look at issues relating to

- research and patenting
- genetic diagnosis and treatment
- screening
- the value and right to know
- responsibility, contributing factors and comorbidity
- privacy and ownership of genetic information:
  - family members
  - employers
  - the police or judiciary
- banking DNA.

We will be especially interested in the ethical, legal and social impacts of knowledge about genetics and what requirements ought to be met by researchers and implementers of this knowledge.

Research and patenting

Case 3
Your health: implications of the human genome project[31]

(From the CNN website, 17 March 2000) As the international research project to decode the DNA within each human cell nears completion,[32] there has been much talk of how the findings of the Human Genome Project will vastly change health care. But what in practical terms are the potential effects on the future of medical therapies and deadly disease?

Among other things, the findings could make it possible to screen children for hundreds of diseases before birth. Genes for an enormous range of traits such as eye and hair color, height, intelligence and longevity may also be known.

It is unlikely a patent will be issued on the gene for a particular eye color. President Clinton and British Prime Minister Tony Blair made it clear in a statement this week that no one should own the information.

But if a couple wanted to change their child's eye color from green to brown, that process could be subject to patent.

While the gene for disease such as cystic fibrosis could not be patented, the therapies developed to treat the disease could be.

CNN Medical Correspondent Rhonda Rowland looks at the implications of these findings, and how pharmaceutical companies are racing to develop therapies which can be patented.

Case 4
Woman files patent application on herself[33]

(Reuters) A British woman has become the first person to attempt to patent herself, the national Patent Office said Tuesday.

'I can confirm that we have received an application with the title "myself" from Donna Rawlinson MacLean,' the Patent Office's Brian Caswell said.

Britain's *Guardian* newspaper said MacLean, a poet and casino waitress from Bristol in the west of England, was angered at the patenting of gene sequences by businesses.

'It has taken 30 years of hard labor for me to discover and invent myself, and now I wish to protect my invention from unauthorized exploitation, genetic or otherwise,' MacLean told the newspaper.

Caswell said the full details of application GB0000180.0 would be published in 18 months.

'It is not really worth patenting something unless you make a lot of money from it,' he added.

Not all stories will seem as bizarre as the above case, but it does illustrate the types of concern the general public have about the nature of genetic research and knowledge or ownership of DNA.

Should we allow the patenting of human genes? Are genes the common property of all humankind, or should the financial rewards of gene research go to individuals and companies who make genetic discoveries?[34]

The above questions will probably be answered in the same way the politicians in Case 3 responded. No one will be permitted to patent genes because they are common to all human beings; it is only their sequencing as DNA that is unique to each individual. What is more likely is that procedures for the identification and manipulation of genetic material will be patented by those innovators who establish them.

This is reassuring because there is a strong sense that the relatively few genes that represent human beings, and indeed all life on this planet, are the common resources and assets of all who share in them. The application of these assets in healthcare treatments is subject to the same social and market forces as any medical treatment. We hope that conditions of justice and beneficence will be applied in their delivery and availability so all humans can have equal access to the type of care genetic discoveries can provide, but there is no doubt that, at some level at least, a profit motive will be involved. Chapter 9 contains a detailed analysis of the ideals of a just healthcare system, the principles of which will apply just as readily to gene therapy.

Genetic diagnosis and treatment

The tests and treatments newly available because of genetic discoveries herald great improvements in the care of individuals suffering from as yet untreatable conditions. There is no doubt of their value to many. Nevertheless, genetic discoveries are not immune to the sorts of ethical problems discussed throughout this book. Some of the problems associated with genetic discoveries

are no different from those associated with any medical practice, although differently applied. Others will be entirely new and therefore new debates, legislation and policy will need to be initiated to ensure that genetics is applied responsibly in health care.

Screening

> **Case 5**
> **Screening for late-onset, as yet incurable, conditions**
>
> Nicole is a 32-year-old married mother of two who works in a plastics factory. Her mother died in her mid-forties after a lengthy battle with breast cancer. On her own initiative and after discussions with her GP and a genetic counsellor, Nicole decides to be tested for the BRCA genes. 'I just want to know one way or the other,' she told the counsellor. 'I have a daughter of my own, and me and my husband – we just want to be prepared. I know there's no real cure right now, but if I know I have the gene I can take precautions.'

Screening for genetic conditions opens a range of difficult ethical challenges for individuals and professional healthcare providers. Case 5 raises these issues so far:

- the value of genetic information and the right to know
- the possible disadvantages of having genetic information
- the impact of genetic information on lifestyle.

The value and right to know

There are obvious benefits to having information about oneself, and especially about one's health. The section about informed consent in Chapter 3 (p. 51) highlights such benefits as the protection of autonomy and freedom to make plans and live one's life coherently and responsibly with the knowledge relevant to doing so. There is little doubt that Nicole will be affected by having knowledge about her

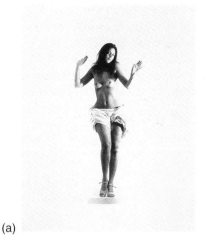

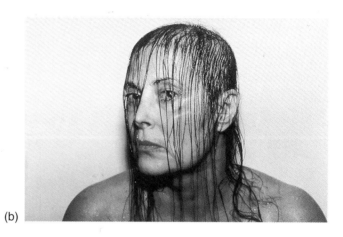

(a)   (b)

Figure 2.2 (a) and (b)
These photographs are of the artist. The first – Super-t-art – was taken long before the second one, from INTRAVENUS which was taken during her illness with a cancer that had killed her mother and ultimately led to her own untimely death. What advantages can there be to knowing how one's genetic inheritance will play itself out? ('Super-t-art' Hannah Wilke 1974 © Estate of Hannah Wilke 2001. Courtesy of Ronald Feldman Fine Arts, New York. Photograph by Christopher Giercke. 'INTRAVENUS' Hannah Wilke 1992 © Estate of Hannah Wilke 2001. Courtesy of Ronald Feldman Fine Arts, New York. Photograph by Dennis Cowley.)

likelihood of developing breast cancer in the future. She has already expressed a belief that she can do something to reduce her risks and make plans accordingly. So increased freedom and respect for autonomy are significant benefits of having genetic information. But not everyone will want to know this information (Fig. 2.2).

The disadvantages of possessing such information are similarly crucial, especially when this means having presymptomatic, personal genetic information about late onset disease for which there is no known cure. This complicated set of concepts is a Pandora's box of concerns. When the condition is presymptomatic there might be little reason for concern, especially where the disease progression is not inevitable in the long run. It is possible that Nicole will become a member of the already overpopulated class of 'worried-well'. These are people who carry with them worries about the possibility of developing illnesses that they might never actually have or which will not affect them for decades. Identifying carriers of

genes does not always mean the individual will inevitably develop the disease, and vice versa. In some cases, such as familial breast cancer, the lifetime likelihood of developing the disease even when one does not carry mutations of one of the breast cancer (BRCA) genes is still in the order of 15%. However, those women who are told they do carry the mutation might worry about developing the disease even more than those who are told they do not carry it. Either way there is a false sense of the realities of developing the condition and the knowledge that one carries the relevant gene may just be a source of unnecessary worry.

A further disadvantage of possessing genetic information is that it could also create a subclass of patients who are not actually ill sometimes known as the 'asymptomatic-ill' or the 'healthy-ill'.[35]

As a large number of individuals submit to or are coerced into genetic testing, in order to obtain employment or insurance cover, a new social class and category – the 'asymptomatic ill' – may be constructed. Although they are healthy, persons in this new group may find that they are treated as if they were disabled or chronically ill by various institutions of our society.[36]

In this case, patients who are not yet affected by a genetically earmarked condition, but who are identified as having the relevant gene, become tied to the notion that they are unwell, even if they are presymptomatic and might never become symptomatic. These people can become subject to prejudice and will be treated as if they were ill, and in some cases act as if they were ill. It is unlikely that most people who will eventually become sufferers of a particular condition will wish to begin their suffering long before any symptoms arise. Here again, the harms of genetic knowledge can be greater than the benefits. The relative harms will probably be mitigated by the inevitability of developing the illness. The greater the likelihood of developing the disease, the greater the likelihood of wanting the information in order to plan for an inevitable decline. But are we sure that everyone would want to know how and when they will die, if they could know in it advance?

On the larger scale, financial issues could become a problem as well. For example, funding for treatment and research into helping those who actually suffer from a condition could be redirected towards the identification and prevention of the condition instead.[37] This might help to resolve some problems, as prevention would theoretically reduce the costs of future care. However, there is no guarantee that prevention will eliminate the condition altogether and some spending and research into cure will still be required.

In the cases of the worried-well and the healthy-ill, the so-called benefits of knowledge about one's own state of health actually become hindrances and appear to reduce the

person's freedom rather than increase it. Beyond that, there will always be competing costs and demands for funds and genetic testing and prevention, all of which will only add to resource problems. As a result of this sort of analysis, we must be drawn to the possibility identified by Sally MacIntyre that, 'we may be introducing tests because they are possible rather than beneficial'.[38]

> Can we be justified in not informing a person that she or he is carrying a gene that will lead to an incurable illness?

Responsibility, contributing factors and comorbidity

> **Case 5 continued…**
> **Contributing factors: nature or nurture?**
>
> Unfortunately, Nicole's test is positive for BRCA2. She is saddened by this information, and struggles with depression for a few weeks. The genetic counsellor points out that she ought to feel empowered by the knowledge, as there are precautionary measures she can take. Nicole, who has always been active, continues her aerobics classes, changes her family's diet and enrols in an aromatherapy course. 'I am taking control of my life' she tells her husband. About a month after her decision she makes an appointment to speak with her GP about the possibility of a prophylactic bilateral radical mastectomy.
>
> In the midst of dealing with all of this, Nicole decides to tell her sister Sheila about the positive test. Nicole tells Sheila that this doesn't mean that Sheila will necessarily carry the genetic mutation, but it is likely. Sheila has four children all under the age of ten. She is a chain smoker and says she barely makes it to the end of each day – never mind exercising – and that she just eats what the kids will eat. 'I have no intention of trying to quit smoking or anything else. If I get cancer I get cancer. It doesn't scare me. I can't start making all those changes now – I just want to live my life.'

In the last section we raised the notion of autonomy and increased freedom related to better knowledge of oneself. We also looked at some ways in which possessing knowledge can reduce freedom. The events described in this part of Nicole and Sheila's case raise new issues related to freedom and autonomy. Does possessing genetic information mean one must act on it? Moreover, do we have the right not to find out what genetic conditions we may be susceptible to?

Nicole has elected to know about her health and to make lifestyle changes accordingly. This could be an expression of autonomy and personal liberty but it could also be described as a restriction to her freedom in the sense of being a hostage to fortunes she can only hope to prevent. No one can force Nicole to choose to make these changes, however much they might help her, but there could be social pressures among other sorts of coercion that guide her down a particular path.

Sheila, on the other hand, wishes not to know and will do nothing to change her own circumstances. Perhaps this is a fatalistic attitude on her part; she might feel there is no point, because, once earmarked for cancer, her situation is hopeless. Can she be condemned for not responding to the possibility that she could reduce her risks by changing her lifestyle?

There are paternalistic and social reasons for criticizing Sheila's choice not to act. After all, there is something she can do to reduce her risk of dying of cancer, so she ought to take these opportunities. From a paternalistic standpoint there could be good reasons for trying to coerce a change in her behaviour and attitude for her own good. From a social perspective, economic factors can be used to criticize her behaviour too. The cost of her healthcare might be higher if she does not respond in the same way her sister does. So justification can be made to ensure she makes changes in order to help keep health costs down (see Chapter 9, p. 171 for more on the question of self-inflicted illness and desert). In addition, her children have a stake in her

behaviour as well. They will benefit from Sheila's improved chance of living a long life without cancer. So it is easy to criticize Sheila's attitude towards having more information about her genetic risks of developing breast cancer. How should she respond to this criticism?

Her first line of defence must surely be that she is an autonomous adult and, as such, must be permitted to act freely in any way she chooses. She can accept offers of help or refuse them. Her actions are primarily selfregarding and, even where they can be shown to interfere with the interests of others (society or her children), she must still be permitted the freedom to act on her own decisions and her right to bodily integrity. She is staking a claim to a right to non-interference, reflective of a belief in tolerance and liberty of the sort supported by John Stuart Mill,[39] who stated that no one has a right to interfere with the self-regarding actions of another person. Where social interests are at stake, Mill would be clear that individual interests must prevail unless a great risk to public safety can be demonstrated (such as the sort of risks aggressive airborne viruses might introduce). There is no such public risk associated with breast cancer, so Sheila can claim to have a right not to find out about her condition and a right not to act on information she may have.

Sheila could also take a different approach. Her response could be to say that she has no control over her genes and that therefore she is no more responsible for her lifestyle choices and behaviour than she is responsible for being susceptible to cancer in the first place.

How will increasing genetic knowledge affect our concepts of freedom and responsibility? To what extent will whole classes of people – from substance abusers to violent criminals – be able to excuse themselves by saying 'My genes made me do it'?[40]

This reveals an added dimension to genetics not discussed so far. There is research evidence to demonstrate that cancer and other illnesses are brought about by several contributing factors, i.e. they are multifactorial. Genes are insufficient causes for the development of cancer. In addition, social and environmental factors contribute to individuals developing the conditions for which they have a genetic predisposition. Should people be held responsible, even though contributing environmental factors may be just as likely to be at fault?

> Clarke has expressed the fear that commercial pressures for susceptibility testing for common disorders 'will promote the notion that the genetic endowment and chosen lifestyle together determine future health, while the importance of material circumstances (especially poverty) in creating ill health will be glossed over.'[41]

The causes of cancer are still not entirely defined. Most of the time, contributing factors complicate the origins of disease, making it impossible to isolate any one cause. Where contributing factors are social, such as poverty and disempowerment, the source and the cure are even more difficult to determine. As a result, the responsibility of Sheila, Nicole and other bearers of cancer genes to do what they can to avoid developing the disease cannot rest solely with them. Social factors have to be addressed as well, but it is not clear that doctors are trained to make these changes. The responsibility therefore, must lie with the community as a whole.

Privacy and ownership of genetic information

One factor we haven't addressed yet is the right of the person to be told about genetic information that could affect them personally. Imagine a situation where Nicole and Sheila had fallen out and had not been on speaking terms for many years. What if Nicole, having discovered that she carried the BRCA gene, decided not to tell Sheila the results? Now, instead of Sheila not wanting to know, Nicole does not want her informed. What rights do Sheila and Nicole have in this situation and what responsibilities does this impose on the doctor?

The law is still debating problems of non-disclosure in this context.[42] No clear solutions have been found. In general, both national[43] and international[44] guidelines prefer to respect individuals' wishes not to know information pertaining to themselves. But the wish not to tell is another problem altogether, and the answer lies, to a great extent, on who the information is going to and why they need to know.[45]

Who ought to have access to genetic information about a particular patient?

- Family members?
- Employers?
- Insurers?
- Police and judiciary?
- Public health registries? (see p. 42 & 129)
- Anyone else?

Family members
In the case of family members, the reasons for wanting the information can be significant enough to place a moral imperative on the individual to disclose information, but only where the:

- risks of not doing so are significant
- potential recipient(s) of the information wish(es) to know.

In cases where the genetically linked illness is likely to emerge, such as Huntington's chorea or muscular dystrophy, there can be significant harms to family members associated with their lack of knowledge. Chief among these is the potential for the gene to be passed on to future generations, a harm that, in some cases, can be avoided (see Chapter 8 on preimplantation screening p. 148). Where the two conditions are satisfied, the onus is on patients to disclose the information themselves. Hopefully they will need little encouragement to do so. If they are reluctant, the responsibility is placed on the doctor or counsellor to try to persuade the patient to disclose the information by pointing out the potential harms and benefits. It is not clear how much effort the healthcare practitioner or the patient ought to put into transferring the information. Problems arise when the patient adamantly refuses to tell certain family members and, more likely, when the patient is not in contact with family members and cannot easily track them down. How far the patient and doctor have to go to discharge their duty to a relative is so far undecided.

Employers

> Case 5 continued...
> **Other concerned parties⁴⁶**
>
> Nicole and Sheila work for Melting's Plastics, Inc., a multinational company with a plastics factory in Millington, north of Glasgow. All the employees in the Manufacturing division have been told in a memo that they will have to reapply for their jobs and submit for genetic screening on application. It was recently discovered that women exposed regularly to certain chemicals in the making of plastic are at 5% increased risk of developing certain forms of cancer, including cervical and breast cancer. All the women working at the plant have been told that they will have to undergo genetic screening and that those found to be carrying high-risk genes will either be offered jobs in a factory near Manchester, which uses a different chemical process, or will not be re-employed.
>   Nicole, Sheila and some of their colleagues are suspicious that this is the company's way of reducing their future losses due to absenteeism by not re-hiring people who have genes linked to a disease or illness that requires extensive time off work. Melting's official notification states 'our primary concern is for the workers'.

Who should have access to our genetic information is most probably best determined on the reason why the information needs to be disclosed. The reason most often supplied is economic. To employers and insurers, the costs of ill-health related to genetic conditions can be great. We can see how it would be in their interest to know who has a predisposition to what sorts of conditions in order to keep the cost of illness low. This is the sort of discrimination most people are afraid will tarnish the excellent help and care genetic information can provide. The application of the information is crucial. Utilitarian application of the sort that promotes economic savings over individual interests is difficult to accept. Any such reasoning would have to be balanced by deontological considerations of human dignity and respect for confidentiality. Not hiring or insuring a person because they carry a particular gene goes against this deontological security. The utilitarian justification is ultimately self-contradictory, at an absurd extreme. As genetic testing becomes more and more advanced, the likely causes of death of most people will eventually be detectable, making employment and insurance impossible for anyone. We are all going to die of something, after all.

In the case of Melting Plastics, Inc., the claim was slightly different. The company said it had the best interest of its employees in mind, trying to protect women at high risk from the effects of the process. If the company is sincere in its concern then there could be sound reasons for permitting the employer to have relevant genetic information about its employees. However, it could be argued that the company's duty to its employees would be sufficiently discharged by informing all applicants of the potential risks and letting them decide for themselves. This would protect informed consent and respect for the employees' autonomy.

The police or judiciary

The next category of interested parties is the police or judiciary. Here the genetic information about a person could be sought to ensure public safety or help to solve a crime. It is not clear to what extent a person ought to be subjected to invasive medical tests to help in a police investigation. The same restrictions discussed in Chapter 8 under bodily integrity would probably apply here. Everyone has a right to privacy and control over their own bodies. We can hope that people would voluntarily help in the event of public risk but they might have reasons not to want to do so. Among these are fear of self-incrimination or unwarranted persecution. These concerns are excellent reasons for prevention of involuntary interference with an individual's life or body. Here a balance between competing interests needs to be negotiated to ensure public safety but not at the expense of uncalled-for individual harm.

Banking DNA

A recent phenomenon in the genetics industry is the emergence of DNA banking facilities. These facilities archive genetic information and store it, at the request of individuals, communities or researchers.

Private DNA banking

The reasons for private individuals to want to save or bank their DNA are probably as numerous as there are people doing it. The advertising in most of the banking facilities suggests the purpose of private DNA banking is to facilitate testing without multiple donations and to help family members to learn about their own genetic status after the death of the person who banks DNA. Future uses could include cloning for implantation of organs and tissue. In this context the DNA is stored privately but the identity of the person storing it is clearly marked, for the purposes of retrieval. This does leave the individual vulnerable to misuse of their DNA, so the specimens are carefully guarded and access to them is restricted to those designated by the owner of the sample. Presumably these samples can be stored for any length of time, even after the death of the originator. Samples will be bequeathed and designated heirs will eventually receive ownership and responsibility of the sample. Insurers and employers, among others, need express permission to access the samples at any time.

Research banks

Research involving human tissue samples is another reason for banking or archiving DNA. Genetic databases derived from a variety of whole populations are stored for access by researchers.[47] Studies into the origins and causes of disease, treatments and other information have provided great benefits to the communities involved and the entire world. The ethical considerations in medical research are addressed in Chapter 7. Special considerations in this context are considered below.

Adequate anonymization
- Samples ought to be stored with a coded marker to ensure privacy
- The number of people with access to the code ought to be confined and regulated.

Adequate consent
- Ensure research participants are aware their DNA samples will be archived and accessed for future research
- Ensure participants have had an opportunity to give valid consent to participate in the current project and if they so chose, to refuse storage and future access by other projects
- An address of the storage facility ought to be provided in case individuals wish to retrieve their samples.

Adequate protection of the samples
- The samples should be well and securely stored
- A person or people ought to be designated the administrator(s) responsible for the stored collection of samples
- Access to the samples for future research ought to be made only on the condition that the new research project has been given full approval by a responsible ethics review committee, such as a Local Research Ethics Committee (LREC) or a Multicentre Research Ethics Committee (MREC) in the UK
- It is important to note that not permitting use of the valuable resource of an archive of samples is problematic. Appropriate use is better than no use at all.

Ownership and benefit rights
- The question of who owns the samples ought to be addressed in advance and proper consent sought
- It might be desirable to allow individuals to retain ownership of their own samples, although what happens to these after the death of the individual would also have to be considered
- Responsibility for the complete set of samples would still be given to the designated administrator to oversee and ensure appropriate usage
- Where possible, the benefits – economic or otherwise – that are derived from the archive ought to be shared with the community of donors as a whole. The share and type of benefit can be worked out in advance and could take the form of access to treatment, sharing in the research findings, education and training and even community improvements.

These are just some reflections to ensure fair and careful practices in genetics research. Many of them are still up for debate and new developments will bring new problems in the future.

Transgenic technology

A final area of interest is the realm of transgenics. This is where the genetic make-up of a creature is manipulated, usually for the purposes of treatment. The most common use of transgenic technology is in xenotransplantation. This topic is addressed in Chapter 5 (p. 102) on ethical issues related to the end of life but it is worth exploring it here in the context of genetics.

Case 6
Xenotransplantation

Rejection hurdle keeps the human factor hypothetical[48]

Alan McDermid, Medical Correspondent

Most of the running on producing pig organs capable of being transplanted to humans has been made by Surrey-based Imutran, a subsidiary of the giant Novartis Group.

It is producing pigs that have normal mothers and fathers but are conceived through IVF and genetically modified at the embryo stage…

Imutran takes a test-tube embryo and micro-injects it with human protein, which is then expressed on the outside of the pig's organs, thereby creating a 'transgenic' pig…

…These measures are aimed at preventing the recipient's immune system from identifying the organ as a foreign body and attacking it.

The creators of the transgenic pig believe they can overcome this hurdle but further rejection remains a long-term threat that may have to be countered by drugs. The other risk is the transfer of some, possibly unknown, organism from the pig that could result in a mutant disease harmful to humans, possibly with the potential to be spread to others.

The most feared is porcine endogenous retrovirus (PERV), which is established in pigs' genes and is inherited by their offspring. Research into this danger is being carried out in Scotland by Q-One Biotech, co-founded by David Onions, Professor of Veterinary Pathology at Glasgow University.

Nevertheless, the UK Xenotransplantation Interim Regulatory Authority is proceeding with caution. As well as monitoring patients, their families and their sexual contacts, it has suggested organ recipients may have to sign an undertaking never to have children.

For those waiting for donor organs, the stakes are high. There were 5396 people waiting for kidney, heart, pancreas, lung and liver transplants at the end of 1999, whereas only 2410 transplants, from 748 donors, were carried out through the year.

Can we ever justify the use of animal organs for the purposes of saving human lives through organ transplantation? Many people believe this is no different to using animals for food. Others say it is better because the result is nobler. Still others say it is a disaster that creates more harm in the long run.

> My view is ethically, we as a community should consider whether or not the costs of going down that route might be heavier than us addressing our own potential responsibility to make sure our organs are used after our death.[49]

This quote places the onus on the community of individuals to donate organs after death so animals do not need to be used for the same purposes. Emerging technologies in cloning have introduced a third option where individual organs will eventually be cloned for the person who needs them. This advance will have the added benefit of removing the requirement for drug treatment to ensure compatibility because the organ would be cloned using DNA from the eventual recipient, making them inherently compatible. Is this an ethically uncontentious use of genetic technology?

Similar genetic manipulation within individual humans raises another area for unease. This is discussed in Chapter 8 (p. 149) where genetic manipulation of fetuses is considered. So far, therapeutic genetic treatment in adults has resulted in the death of one patient. Experiments persist but break-throughs are slow. It raises fears of genetic manipulation for social factors as well as clinical conditions. We might be able to improve therapeutic options for people with genetically linked conditions such as breast cancer, cystic fibrosis or muscular dystrophy. However, how far we will permit genetic manipulation is debatable. The possibilities seem endless from here, especially when behavioural links to genetics enter the picture. Will it be permissible to alter the DNA of repeat criminal offenders who have violent tendencies? How about choosing to alter your sense of humour? Will genetic manipulation become just another form of plastic surgery in a world where personal augmentation and transformation is already an accepted norm? Only time will tell.

Conclusion

This chapter introduced a number of significant issues related to patient care and the responsibilities conferred upon doctors. The issues explored here will be revisited in future chapters, where relevant. It will be useful to keep in mind the material discussed so far when making consideration of the rest of the material covered in this book. Ideas to keep in mind are:

- the details of professional behaviour
- the importance of good communication skills
- issues related to team delivery of healthcare
- advocacy and the duties of professional healthcare providers
- patients with special needs
- the impact of genetics on clinical relationships.

Notes and references

1 Tomorrow's Doctors. London: GMC 1993.
2 New Doctor. London: GMM 1997.

3 For a very clear discussion of this subject see Downie R, Calman K. Healthy respect: ethics in health care. 2nd ed. Oxford: Oxford University Press; 1994.

4 Belbin RM. Team roles at work. Oxford: Butterworth Heinemann 1993.

5 Ritter S. Does the team work? Nursing Times 1984.

6 Schwartz L. Is there an advocate in the house? The role of Health Care Professionals in patient advocacy. J Medical Ethics 2002; 28:0–3.

7 Professional guidance has highlighted these and similar responsibilities. For example, see General Medical Council. Good medical practice. London: GMC Publications; July 1998.

8 See: Willard C. The nurse's role as patient advocate – obligation or imposition. J Adv Nursing 1996; 24:60–66 and Caplan A. The ethics of gatekeeping in rehabilitation medicine. J Head Trauma Rehab 1997; 12:29–36.

9 See: Burke MJ. Clinicoeconomics in geropsychiatry. Psychiatr Clin N Am 1997; 20:219 and Caplan A. The ethics of gatekeeping in rehabilitation medicine. J Head Trauma Rehab 1997; 12:29–36 and Hazzard WR. Elder abuse – definitions and implications for medical education. Academic Med 1995; 70:979–981.

10 Saiki-Craighill S. The children's sentinels: mothers and their relationships with health professionals in the context of Japanese health care. Soc Sci Med 1997; 44:291–300.

11 Haberfellner EM, Rittmannsberger H. Involuntary admission at psychiatric hospitals – the situation in Austria. Psychiatrische Praxis 1996; 23:139–142.

12 See: Bloche GM. Fidelity and deceit at the bedside. JAMA 2000; 283:1181 and Rosner F. The ethics of managed care. Mount Sinai J Med 1997; 64:8–19.

13 Faherty B. Now is the time to advocate. Nursing Outlook 1993; 41:248–249.

14 Esterhuizen P. Is the professional code still the cornerstone of clinical nursing practice? J Adv Nursing 1996; 23:25–31.

15 United Kingdom Central Council of Nursing. Code of professional conduct. London: UKCC; June 1992.

16 Burke MJ. Clinicoeconomics in geropsychiatry. Psychiatr Clin N Am 1997; 20:219.

17 Willard C. The nurse's role as patient advocate – obligation or imposition. J Adv Nursing 1996; 24:60–66.

18 Willard C. The nurse's role as patient advocate – obligation or imposition. J Adv Nursing 1996; 24:60–66.

19 Faherty B. Now is the time to advocate. Nursing Outlook 1993; 41:248–249.

20 Berlandi JLH. Ethical issues in paediatric preoperative nursing. Nursing Clin N Am 1997; 32:153.

21 See: Bird AW. Enhancing patient well-being – advocacy or negotiation. J Medical Ethics 1994, 20:152–156 and Willard C. The nurse's role as patient advocate – obligation or imposition. J Adv Nursing 1996; 24:60–66.

22 Mallik M. Advocacy in nursing – a review of the literature. J Adv Nursing 1997; 25:130–138.

23 Hazzard WR. Elder abuse – definitions and implications for medical education. Academic Med 1995; 70:979–981.

24 Age of Legal Capacity (Scotland) Act 1991.

25 Family Law Reform Act 1969.

26 *Good Practice in consent implementation guide* Department of Health 2001.

27 Dickenson D. Children's informed consent to treatment: is the law an ass? J Medical Ethics 1994; 20:205–206.

28 Details of what Jehovah's Witnesses believe about blood transfusion are available on the British Medical Journal website (http://www.bmj.com). Select the search/archive option and type 'Jehovah' in the 'Words in the title' option.

29 Adults with Incapacity (Scotland) Act 2000.

30 Skelton P. Pamela Hurwitz and her friends, exhibition and book. ARTicle Press; Broadside series number 6, January 2001.

31 CNN Your Health. Available: http://cnn.com/2000/HEALTH/03/17/genome.proj ect/index.html 17 March 2000. Web posted at: 12:40 p.m. EST (1740 GMT).

32 It may be of interest that the decoding was completed just a few months after this article was published.

33 Oddly Enough Headlines. Available: http://dailynews.yahoo.com/htx/nm/20000229/od/ patent_1.html Tuesday 29 February 2000 8:41 a.m. EST

34 Available: http://www.dartmouth.edu/artsci/ethics-inst/application1.html#course

35 Hubbard R. Predictive genetics and the construction of the healthy-ill. Suffolk University Law Review 1993; 1209:1212–1220.

36 Billings et al Discrimination as a consequence of genetic testing. Am J Hum Genet 1992; 50:476–482.

37 MacIntyre S. Social and psychological issues associated with the new genetics. Phil Trans R Soc London B 1997; 352:1095–1101.

38 MacIntyre S. Social and psychological issues associated with the new genetics. Phil Trans R Soc London B 1997; 352:1095–1101.

39 Mill JS. On liberty. Indianapolis: Bobbs-Merrill. 1956.

40 Available: http://www.dartmouth.edu/artsci/ethics-inst/application1.html#course

41 Clarke A. Population screening for genetic susceptibility to disease. Br Med J 1996; 311:35–38 as quoted in MacIntyre S. Social and psychological issues associated with the new genetics. Phil Trans R Soc London B 1997; 352:1095–1101.

42 Laurie GT. Wielding the implement of law: distilling new rights and responsibilities in the age of the 'new genetics'. Health, Risk and Society 1999; 1(3):333–341.

43 The Human Genetics Advisory Commission 1997; British Medical Association 1998 and the Nuffield Council on Bioethics 1993.

44 UNESCO Universal Declaration on the Human Genome and Human Rights, available at: http://www.unesco.org/ethics; and The Council of Europe Convention for the Protection of Human Rights and Dignity of the Human Being with regard to the Application of Biology and Medicine, available at http://www.legal.coe.int/bioethics/gb/html/txt_adopt.htm.

45 Balint J. Issues of privacy and confidentiality in the new genetics. Albany Law J Sci Technol 1998; 9:27–38.

46 Based on a case from The Human Genome Project: Exploring the Scientific and Humanistic Dimensions website developed by the Massachusetts Corporation for Educational Telecommunications (MCET). Available: http://www.mcet.edu/genome/issuesandethics/forum/dec2/forum.html

47 For example, see Mapping the Icelandic Genome project. Available: http://sunsite.berkeley.edu/biotech/iceland/

48 McDermid A. The Herald. Wednesday 15 March 2000; 14.

49 Professor Sheila McLean, quoted in The Herald. Wednesday 15 March 2000; 14.

3

Rights of patients, practitioners and society

In Chapter 1, rights theory was loosely described. Chapter 2 highlighted some of the duties expected of medical professionals. This chapter examines the rights of patients and corresponding duties they impose on practitioners. Beginning with an analysis of the bearing the United Nations Declaration of Human Rights has on medical practice, and detailed examination of two of the most important rights often ascribed to patients, namely the right to confidentiality and the right to give or withhold consent. This will be followed by brief explorations of the rights of practitioners and the rights of society.

Rights of patients

The Universal Declaration of Human Rights (Appendix 2) was published in 1948. Although the Declaration embraces the rights of primarily 'fit' humans, part of its motivation was the phenomenon of experimentation by medical doctors on non-consenting, even constrained, persons. The following aspects of the Declaration bear on medical practice.

> Article 1. Because all human beings are born free and equal in dignity and rights, they should act as brothers towards each other.

This concept implies that brothers behave well and honourably and morally towards each other, which, unfortunately, we know from the Bible (Genesis 4.8) has not happened since the beginning of time. Clearly what is intended here, and what is relevant for the doctor, is the meaning that each human should treat all others with respect,

for practical purposes, as one would wish to be treated oneself.

The New Testament resumé of the Torah summarizes the spirit of Article 1, namely, 'You shall love your neighbour as yourself' (John 13.34).

> Article 2. No distinction should be made determined by colour, nationality, politics, possessions, race, religion, sex, or status.

Doctors need constantly to be careful not to discriminate in any way as they go about their lives managing patients, who will display an infinite variety of these above listed characteristics. It is worryingly easy to favour some individuals, possibly because they are neighbours or belong to some group to which we are affiliated.

> Article 3. Everyone has the right to life, liberty and security of person.

Clearly, 'the right to life' is fundamental to the doctor, whose job is frequently to maintain, or even save, the lives of patients. Consideration of what life is, and of its quality and possible sanctity, is given in Chapter 6, as are issues such as when maintenance of life is desirable, and when this is futile. 'Liberty' and 'security' are the other two components of this Article. As far as possible, doctors must also give these rights to their patients. Ways in which a doctor might fail in these areas include detaining patients longer than their management strictly requires (for example, to ensure that hospital beds are available for patients on scheduled operating lists, surgeons sometimes 'block' beds to prevent emergency cases being admitted before the elective patients have arrived) and by failing to protect fellow patients from one who was violent or dangerous. (Note, however, that effecting security for the safety of the greater number of patients could mean depriving the individual regarded as dangerous of liberty).

> Article 4. No one shall be held in servitude or slavery.

Although it is unlikely that a doctor might do these things to patients, one circumstance in which doctors can effectively enslave people is colleagues – particularly juniors – by setting demands and standards for medical work in settings where resources are short and long hours are required from members of the healthcare team. To some extent, the neglect of this human right for healthcare professionals is a regular feature of government-funded health services, although recent legislation is attempting to address excessive hours of work in Europe.

> Article 5. No one shall be subjected to torture, degrading treatment or punishment.

Observing this Article might be difficult for doctors who work for the state, particularly in those countries where capital punishment is the law.[1] For, by being present, a doctor can ensure that the condemned individual is executed in a way in which physical suffering is reduced to the minimum. Similar arguments apply to medical personnel attending interrogation procedures, which might be deemed necessary to maintain law and order but that might be 'degrading' or even torturous.

> Articles 6, 7, 8, 9, 10 and 11. No one shall be disenfranchised of law…

When patients are recruited to participate in medical research, doctors must remember that these patients must not be denied this basic human right to redress from the law of the land. In the desire to find cures for cruel diseases, doctors can be tempted to minimize, or even neglect, this right of their patients to participate voluntarily, and to withdraw whenever they wish without explanation.

> Article 12. Everyone has the right to privacy of correspondence, family and home. Honour nor reputation should be attacked.

Confidentiality is paramount for doctors in their dealings with patients. This is so important that, in practice, it is safer to err on the side of being over discreet. A tension with this article arises in relation to epidemiology and public health, particularly in the context of clinical and molecular genetics. Both society and the profession of medicine need to enhance knowledge of health and disease. One of the ways in which these objectives were most effectively achieved during the twentieth century was by death certification and registers of particular diseases, such as cancer registries (see p. 34). Currently, predisposition to particular inheritable diseases in individuals and their families is pursued by linking information in a family tree. It is not uncommon for people who trace their genealogy to be unpleasantly surprised by information they discover about their ancestors. Currently, legislators are concerned to protect the confidentiality of data such as the identity of forebears and registered causes of death. This legislative initiative is trying to outlaw disease registration, such as national cancer registries. In a democracy, where legislation is implemented by individuals elected by the people, this might happen. However, before it does, the general public should have had the opportunity to think about the consequences. The gains made, by way of enhanced privacy, have to be balanced with the losses incurred both for individuals and for medical scientific research.

> Article 13. Everyone has the right of freedom of movement.

This right is one that doctors may, in the course of their professional duties, need to deny to some patients. This is likely to arise in the context of patients acquiring infectious diseases, which can be spread to other individuals and to whole communities by an infected individual travelling. For most infectious diseases, the time period when the condition is transmissible is limited. For those infectious diseases where effective methods of immunization exist, it makes sense to delay the travel of an infected individual into a community that is vulnerable but that could be rendered immune in a relatively short time by an immunization programme.

Articles 14 and 15 concern asylum and nationality. These articles have little medical relevance.

> Article 16. Everyone has the right to marry and procreate.

This article is also one that medical reasoning might oppose for the good of society at large or for the wellbeing of potential offspring. There are a number of classic examples of these. Huntington's chorea (Saint Vitus' dance) is an inherited condition that affects adults, causing them to have involuntary movements and progressive intellectual impairment, such that affected individuals become completely unable to look after themselves, usually dying about 15 years after the onset of the disease. In addition to the premature death, the protracted period of dying is profoundly unpleasant to the affected individual, as well as to relatives and friends. As the mode of inheritance is dominant, 50% of the offspring of an affected individual will themselves be affected. The physical and psychological nature of this condition is such that most doctors (and, indeed, many members of society) consider it better for carriers of Huntington's chorea not to procreate.

> Is this fair? What are your views?

> Article 17. No one shall be arbitrarily deprived of the right to own property.

Although doctors are unlikely, in the course of professional duties, to want to stop their patients owning property, doctors often need to persuade, even to require, patients who are intellectually or physically impaired, to give up their homes when their disabilities make them a danger to themselves and to others.

> Article 18. Everyone has the right to freedom to observe and practise religion.

In the later part of the twentieth century, doctors in a number of contexts were known to have actively opposed this Article. Such opposition tends to happen when the practice of a religious observance results in damage being done to adherents or their families. A frequently cited example of this concerns ritual circumcision, especially of females. Western medicine regards excision of the external genitalia as depriving the recipients of normal pleasurable experiences, as well as making childbirth unnecessarily difficult and dangerous.

> Article 19. Everyone has the right to hold opinions and impart ideas without interference.

Like Article 18, this Article requires some important modifications to be accepted by doctors. The ideal of freedom of speech is desirable for doctors but they would want to ensure that dangerous delusional ideas (such as those of the Jonestown group, members of which believed that the end of the world was at hand and, *en masse*, ended their own lives) were constrained and not promulgated by any medium and across all boundaries.

> Articles 20 and 21. These concern participation in political activities.

Doctors are unlikely to want to prevent their patients participating in political activities. However, it is just possible to imagine a doctor who finds a patient's political views so vehemently opposed to his or her own that he or she modifies the advice or treatment given to the patient in an attempt to inhibit the patient's participation in political activity.

Article 22. Every one has the right to social security.

The opinions of doctors are often relied upon in relation to claims for pecuniary social security support. Many doctors would consider that economic, personality and social development are the responsibility, rather than the right, of the individual.

Articles 23 to 30. These deal with rights to work, remuneration, leisure, education and culture.

Doctors will acquiesce with a concluding statement that free and full development is only possible by individuals recognizing and exercising their own duties to their communities. For healthcare professionals, this is the duty to care.

Confidentiality

Case 7
The family

Mrs Goldberg is a 43-year-old scriptwriter. She has recently noticed strange symptoms, which have been diagnosed as early symptoms of multiple sclerosis. She realizes she could be relatively unaffected by the disease for some time and so has asked her GP not to tell anyone, not even her family. Mrs Goldberg is married to a computer consultant and has three children, Cathy aged 19, Lara aged 16 and Carl aged 12. The entire family has been under the care of the same general practice since they moved to the area 14 years earlier. Shirley Dawson, the GP, believes she has a good relationship with the Goldbergs, having looked after them through pregnancy, childhood diseases and minor ailments. She is torn by Mrs Goldberg's decision because she feels it would be better for the family if they knew now rather than finding out later. When Shirley asks why Mrs Goldberg wants to keep this secret, Mrs G. explains that 'this would put a strain on all of them. Besides, I don't want them to start treating me differently. I want to look after my family for as long as I can before they start looking after me.'

Confidentiality is among the most persistently acknowledged topics in medical ethics. Normally, theorists do not contest its importance and it is recorded in legal documents and the codes and regulations published by professional bodies. On the surface, cases such as the one above do not present particularly challenging problems to preserving patient confidentiality. A patient requests privacy regarding her own physical condition. A competent and reasonable person makes the request. She supplies a coherent and meaningful explanation for her decision. The disease is in its early stages and does not generally prevent its sufferers from making informed choices for themselves. All in all, there does not appear to be any reason for denying that Mrs Goldberg is in an adequate frame of mind for making the autonomous choice not to inform her family of her condition.

Nevertheless, when we try to relate the situation to a real-life course of events, small doubts begin to emerge regarding the suitability of the patient's decision to keep this information from her family. And, although it is not the doctor's place to disclose information to family members of patients in Mrs Goldberg's position, it is also true that the doctor could be uncomfortable with agreeing to let her endure such a difficult experience without family support. Professional healthcare deliverers are encouraged to empathize with their patients and an understanding of this patient's position, coupled with experience of other similar cases, might make Dr Dawson uncomfortable about not telling a caring family this significant information. Still, there is little disagreement that physicians *cannot* disclose information to family and friends of patients no matter how profound and genuine their concerns. Doing so without prior patient permission is a breach of the doctor–patient relationship and will damage the trust between them. Instead, Dr Dawson would probably try to gently persuade Mrs Goldberg to reconsider her decision, suggesting that the support of her family will be invaluable to her just now. She might also argue that family members could react adversely to discovering later on that such a significant life event was withheld from them. Knowing sooner rather than later would give them time to adjust and prepare themselves, as well as make the most of the best times they have left together. Although, any number of emotive and practical rationalisations could be made to persuade the patient to change her mind, in the end the GP is bound by professional obligations to maintain the patient's confidentiality.

Dr Dawson's conflict regarding maintaining her patient's confidentiality is a very real experience for professional healthcare providers. Professionals might encounter even more firmly established reasons for breaching patient confidentiality. Because of this conflict, it is not satisfactory simply to say that the law and professional codes make confidentiality necessary, without exploring the reasons why it is so important in the therapeutic relationship. These reasons are many and varied; we will examine some of them in an attempt to provide a closer analysis of the case above, and follow with discussion of two further cases that represent strong counterclaims to maintaining confidentiality under all conditions. As we will see, even the law is ambivalent about the sanctity of the confidentiality in some cases.

The requirement of confidentiality is founded on several important elements that will be examined in turn. They include:

1. Protection of privacy:
   – creation and control of one's self identity
   – protection and respect for patient autonomy
2. Trust between patient and care provider:
   – the importance of candour in the therapeutic relationship.

The advantages of confidentiality

Identity, privacy and autonomy. There is an often-ignored aspect for the need for personal privacy that helps explain the importance of protecting patient confidentiality. This is a philosophical concept based on the creation of personal identity. According to some theorists, people create their identities through the information they disclose to others, balanced by the information they withhold. People know, form opinions about and value other people based on information they possess about those people. Thus, the more people can restrict what others know about them, the more they will be able to control the image others have of them, although they will never have complete control over this image, as others extrapolate from what they know and will also observe or learn things the individuals have not disclosed intentionally. Nevertheless, the command people have over the opinion of others can withstand complete overpowering if they withhold certain important aspects of their character or life experiences. Those to whom they disclose more information will have a better understanding of their identity.

Control over the information others have of us can be the only way we have to influence their perceptions of us. Thus, it is imperative that individuals decide for themselves what they do and do not want others to know about them. This can be especially significant in the area of healthcare. Take Mrs Goldberg, for example (see p. 44). She might want to ensure that she can continue her identity as mother and spouse without being affected by her family's reaction to knowledge of her illness. She insists that 'I don't want them to start treating me differently', because she is concerned that knowledge of her condition will change their image of her and she will lose control over her identity as they see it. So maintaining her confidentiality, as she requests, is in part so that she can protect her family's perception of her identity – their interpretation of who she is.

By helping the patient maintain control over information others have of her the practitioner is also helping to preserve and respect the patient's autonomy. Mrs Goldberg will be able to continue living the way she chooses without letting others interfere with this. She will be able to carry on working as a script writer and carry on leading her relationships without interference from others. Provided her illness does not become a hazard to others, it will be the duty of the doctor to allow her to make this choice, and all other self-regarding choices. Only in this way can the patient continue to be autonomously self-governing and self-determining. If the patient loses control of her privacy regarding the intimate details of her personal life, she loses the dignity of her personal autonomy. Moreover, confidentiality protects the individual's right of property over information known about themselves. In this way respect for confidentiality shows respect for persons.

Trust and the importance of candour in the therapeutic relationship

> Without assurances about confidentiality patients may be reluctant to give doctors the information they need in order to provide good care.[2]

The therapeutic relationship relies heavily on patients feeling comfortable to disclose information to their caregivers. Patients might disclose information to their doctors and nurses that they would not tell anyone else, not even their life partners and closest friends. Disclosure of information is in part necessary because trying to provide adequate diagnosis and treatment without the relevant information can be difficult or even impossible. Imagine if Mrs Goldberg had decided not to reveal some vital piece of information about her condition, withholding it because she did not trust her doctor to keep the information from her family or friends. This would complicate matters substantially and a delay in receiving information would mean a delay in providing proper care for Mrs Goldberg.

Patients can choose not to reveal any number of conditions or symptoms that will delay proper care and affect their choices for treatment later on. We can imagine an even worse scenario where a female adolescent, consulting for what appears to be a simple upset stomach, does not trust her doctor enough to reveal that she has been sexually active and missing her periods. Delay of accurate diagnosis of a pregnancy will eliminate the teenager's choices later on, and complicate matters further. We could argue that delays due to lack of disclosure would hurt only the patient herself, but this is not necessarily the case. Lack of information would prolong diagnosis, creating demands for more, sometimes expensive, diagnostic treatments, and possibly mean providing inappropriate therapy for the patient. All of this would be a waste of valuable resources and have indirect impact on the community as a whole. Add to this the possible hardships incurred by the patient, her family and others to whom she is responsible and it looks as if what is superficially only a self-regarding decision, has impact beyond the harm it can cause to the individual patient.

These examples illustrate distinct support for the importance of patient candour and honesty in the therapeutic relationship. Thus, trust between the patient and doctor can be taken to be a necessary aspect of care, and not just an ideal. Maintaining confidentiality is one of the more important elements in preserving that trust.

Patients might be expected to share information about themselves that they would not discuss with anyone else. To maintain this candour and trust, it is imperative that patients are assured that the information they share with their physician will not be passed on to anyone without good cause. Patients also want to be assured that information they share with their doctor will not be made known to anyone else without their permission. Some will enquire about this before they disclose information, although more often it is assumed by the patient and should be taken as understood by the doctor even when the patient does not request it directly. However, there are some important exceptions, as we shall see, and it is imperative that patients be informed in advance of the disclosure when a professional anticipates that it will be necessary to breach a patient's confidence.

Exceptions to confidentiality

Now we can consider some of the exceptions to confidentiality and arguments in favour of disclosure in certain circumstances. The following case study offers one very serious challenge to the primacy of patients' confidentiality:

Case 8
Risky behaviour

Dr Stone's last appointment of the day was with Maureen Cullen, a 32-year-old patient. Maureen is an intravenous heroin user and Dr Stone has treated her for related complications over the last 5 years. He had succeeded, with effort, in helping Maureen to cut back her using and find a council flat. This visit, Maureen was complaining of a cough that 'just hasn't let me be for 3 or 4 weeks, an' an awful sore throat doctor.' On examination, Dr Stone was concerned to note that Maureen's chest was not clear on auscultation and her throat and tongue revealed a white coating with a pink swollen sore. Aware that Maureen had shared needles in the past, and uncertain whether she had indeed stopped doing so in spite of the clean needle exchange run by the health centre, Dr Stone gently suggests to Maureen that this may be related to something more serious. He tells Maureen that he would like to run further tests, and discusses the possibility that she may have HIV. Maureen appeared shaken but not surprised by this suggestion and confides that she has wondered about the possibility when a friend with whom she had shared needles died of AIDS last summer. Maureen gives her consent to an HIV test and Dr Stone asks her to return in a fortnight and to promise not to share any needles or have any unprotected sex until they know for certain what is causing her illness.

Three days later Dr Stone sees a new patient in his surgery. Lindsey is a 29-year-old unemployed single woman. She tells Dr Stone that she has just moved to the neighbourhood and her new flatmate, Maureen Cullen, suggested he would add her to his register. On discussion, Lindsey reveals that she is also an intravenous heroin user, but what concerns Dr Stone even more is that she tells him that she and Maureen occasionally share needles.

This case presents a problem for the doctor and a serious challenge to the primacy of protecting patient confidentiality. It is not the only sort of situation that promotes these doubts, but it is an important one that cannot be overlooked. It is because of cases such as this that there are times when information can or will be divulged. We will consider the exceptions to confidentiality at the same time as we explore this case.

Times when a medical professional might feel a need to breach patient confidentiality include:

- when the patient is a danger to herself
- in the best interest of the community or a third party
- when required to by the police or judiciary or when ordered to do so by a court
- when prior permission is granted by the patient
- with prior permission to employers and insurance companies
- within a care-providing team or when consulting healthcare colleagues
- for the purpose of research, teaching or audit

Danger to self. A healthcare professional might find it necessary to breach patient confidentiality in situations where a patient intends to self-harm, such as suicide or self-mutilation. In such cases, the professional must be very careful to inform only those who could truly be of help to the patient. However, the situation can backfire if, by informing on the patient, the doctor destroys the trust they have built up between them. If this happens, patients could resist help in the future or refrain from telling the doctor their plans, making it impossible for the doctor to be of any help.

Danger to others and the community. In Case 8, a conflict arises between protecting the privacy of the patient and protecting the health of another person (or persons). It is further complicated because the second person is also Dr Stone's patient and therefore is owed the same duty of care as the first patient. But determining which patient's interests will come first is not at all simple. On the contrary, this case presents the physician with an impossible situation to resolve without doing harm to one or the other of his patients. The General Medical Council advise that where the benefits to an individual or society of the disclosure outweigh the public and the patient's interest in keeping information confidential, disclosure without consent may be justified. Where you believe patients to be the victims of neglect or abuse and unable to give consent you should inform an appropriate person or agency if you believe it is in the patient's best interests.

Comparing a deontological and a consequentialist perspective. Assuming a deontological perspective of this case does not make the situation any easier. The deontologist will assume a duty to care for patients and protect them from harm, but does this mean protecting the first patient from the harm of a breach to her confidentiality or protecting the second patient from the potential harm of contracting HIV? The answer to this is not obvious. Especially when we compare knowledge of a certain harm with knowledge of only a potential harm.

Nor does consequentialism provide any distinct solution to the matter. The consequences of a breach to Maureen's confidentiality do protect Lindsey from harm; however the breach is also likely to cause Maureen to lose confidence in Dr Stone and set up enough mistrust to prevent her from seeking his, or any, further help. If she is HIV positive but does not know about it or seek proper management, care and treatment then she risks harming herself and others besides Lindsey. So Dr Stone is caught in a position where anything he does will produce some harm to his patients and others.

There is precarious agreement among theorists that the good of the individual patient can be forfeited where the good of others or the good of the community are at stake. This means that confidentiality can be breached and other freedoms that patients expect can be legitimately curtailed if doing so will prevent some serious harm to the community or to a member of the community. Real case examples of this situation are not uncommon. Significant among them are the case of 'Typhoid Mary' who was held for treatment against her will to protect the community from her spreading the disease she carried. Other cases involve involuntary treatment for tuberculosis, reporting a person with epilepsy to traffic control authorities and, most importantly, the Tarasoff case in the US.[3] In all these cases the good of the community was given precedence over the good of the individual and ensuing violations were justified in this way. However, many harbour doubts about the primacy of the community over that of the individual. Their claim is that individuals need protection from the tyranny of the collective as it is represented by society or a community of other individuals. In the case of typhoid Mary, for example, one author argues that Mary Mallon's involuntary incarceration was a violation of her rights and that she should have been allowed to refuse the uncomfortable treatment to which she was forced to submit, just as any patient is allowed to do.[4] For the same reason, the breach of confidentiality required to protect unwitting participants of needle sharing with Maureen Cullen can be seen as an unjustifiable violation of Maureen's rights. It is unclear whether undetermined others deserve the same protection that a determined individual deserves because the faceless others cannot be said to demand their right to be protected, whereas the individual can. From this perspective, Maureen's right to confidentiality ought to be preserved at any cost because she is one actual person confronted by the threat of the 'the mob'. On the other hand, Dr Stone is not considering a faceless mob but an actual other patient to whom he owes a duty of care. As a result, in this case the right of Maureen to have her confidentiality protected is not at all clear, as we have seen.

Police and the judiciary. It is generally accepted that a doctor must disclose information if ordered to do so by a court. However disclosures of information without a patient's consent to the police could only be justified if a failure to do so would hinder the prevention, detection or prosecution of serious crime such as murder or rape. Interference with the course of a legal investigation is sanctioned as well. It is up to the conscience of the individual practitioner to decide whether it is worth facing the sanctions in a particular case and defending the patient's confidentiality in spite of possible punishment.

Failure to prevent a crime can result in a healthcare worker being held liable, as it was in the Tarasoff case. Here, the University of California student health centre was successfully sued by the family for failing to inform Ms Tarasoff of a patient's intention to harm her. A psychologist was aware of this intention but did not warn Ms Tarasoff because he did not want to break his patient's confidentiality. The patient murdered Ms Tarasoff and the psychologist was sued, leaving the way open for practitioners to break confidentiality in similar situations in the US. Indeed, the case has opened the way for like requirements in many countries.[5]

With patient permission. Normally, any breach of confidentiality will be discussed with the patient in advance, and permission sought from the patient to disclose the relevant information. In Case 8, Dr Stone could try to discuss the situation with Maureen and attempt to persuade her that if she refuses to stop sharing needles she should at least inform the person she shares with that she might be HIV positive. He can make these, hopefully

persuasive, arguments without mentioning Lindsey specifically, thereby preserving her confidentiality as well. Dr Stone can attempt to convince Maureen that disclosure would be best for all concerned and, if this didn't work, could inform her that he would find it necessary to breach her confidentiality in order to protect another patient. Then, if she refused to inform Lindsey herself, at least Maureen would have been warned that the information would be disclosed against her wish for the protection of another. In this way Dr Stone can be seen to be carrying out his duty of care to both patients.

Other circumstances for seeking permission to disclose patient information are in the case where the police or judiciary requests it, or when it is requested by an employer or insurance company. Then the doctor must seek explicit permission from the patient and explain in advance what information will be imparted. It must be noted that not all information needs to be revealed. Only information directly related to the request being made ought to be disclosed, and the patient needs to be aware of this as well.[6]

Colleagues and teams. Disclosure between colleagues and among teams can be argued for primarily because it is to the benefit of the patient. Ordinary advice-seeking from colleagues is usually accepted, and even expected, by patients. Nevertheless, it does require discretion from the doctor. Withholding the name of the patient is a simple enough way to ensure that privacy is maintained. In addition, care ought to be taken that the patient's identity is not disclosed accidentally by divulging too much information or aspects of the case that are extraordinary or unique. These ought to be disclosed only when necessary for helping the patient directly or when patient permission is granted for teaching purposes. Also, care should be taken regarding the time and place these discussions are held. Elevator gossip and conversations over lunch can be easily overheard by (un)concerned parties and the patient's privacy unwittingly breached. These commonsense precautions are simple ways of preserving the patient's trust.

New complications have begun to arise in the team care setting. In this situation, patients might disclose information to one member of the team but not to the others. They might even stipulate that they do not wish other members of the team to find out. In this case it is best for the team members to inform the patient in advance that they might be unable to keep the information confidential if they believe it is not in the best interest of the patient to do so. However, they can promise to disclose the information only to relevant team members rather than the entire team. In this way the patient has advance warning of the possible breach and can elect not to share the information. On the other hand, team members might feel it is important that the information be shared anyway, because secrecy can be as detrimental to care as the loss of trust. In such cases, the caregivers are in a difficult position and must consider how best to maintain their duty of care of the patient. Generally speaking, it ought to be made clear to the patient from the outset that team approaches to healthcare require full disclosure within the team, that this is for the good of the patient and that confidentiality will be preserved outside the team.

Records. Permission to view patients' records is another area of concern for confidentiality. This will be considered in more depth in relation to ethical issues in research (Chapter 7, p. 129). However, the following case illustrates the difficulties involved in a similar situation.

Case 9
Homework assignment

A medical student assigned to your practice is found looking at a patient's file without asking permission to do so. When confronted she responds 'I didn't realize I needed to ask, I was just doing an assignment that requires us to report on the medical history of a patient.'

There are two perspectives one can take on this case: (i) the student's behaviour is acceptable because it is part of a homework assignment; or (ii) the student's behaviour is an unacceptable breach of confidentiality. Part of the difficulty in this case is that there are good arguments to support the use of patient records in educational contexts. Chief among these is that students gain valuable experience from viewing actual case records, just as they benefit from examining actual patients. They can be taught through models but, at some point, they need to have experience of the real thing. This can be said to be of benefit to patients because the students will be better educated if they work on real-life records. Some even argue that we have a duty to permit this kind of educational practice and submit to it because it is for the best interest of the community in the long run, and ourselves as members of the community, if students are educated in the best way possible. The same can be said of research and audit practices that will eventually benefit the community. On the other hand, the medical student did not ask permission to explore a patient's record. It is possible that, had she done so, precautions could have been taken to protect confidentiality by hiding the name and address of the patient, as well as other information not relevant to the project.

Access to patient records might be useful and even necessary for educational and other purposes but this does not mean that students and researchers need access to complete records. However, it can take time and effort to alter records to preserve confidentiality and this can take valuable time from patient care. To help alleviate this burden, the patient's permission could be sought beforehand. Again, however, this could involve the time and effort of detailed discussions. To avoid this, patients could be made aware at a first appointment that students and researchers might view their records, and their permission or refusal recorded in their records in advance. Furthermore, students, teachers and researchers need to be aware that educational forays and research initiatives into patient files are a violation of patient privacy. If this is absolutely necessary, then it is best to ensure that they have permission to use the records in the first place.[7]

Summary

In conclusion, information divulged by patients to professional healthcare providers is information that belongs to that patient. The delivery of healthcare depends upon information sharing and, for this reason, confidentiality requires discretion. This means that it might not be exclusive, but that careful consideration must be given before divulging any information about a patient, whether that be to a fellow team member, a consulting colleague or a friend outside work. Careful precautions and considerations of the importance of confidentiality for the reasons described in this chapter will ensure the best care is given to patients and respect for their personhood maintained.

Consider the following questions:

- Why do people need to keep control of the information people know about them? What are the advantages and disadvantages of this?
- When would a healthcare professional feel the need to breach confidentiality and what are the advantages and disadvantages of doing so?

Consent

Another area of medical ethics that generates a great deal of consensus is the importance of obtaining consent from patients before performing any procedure involving them. The agreement over its importance does not, however, lessen the disputes attached to its application or description.

Informed consent can be portrayed with two broad points:

1. The right of a reasonably competent person to make a decision to permit or refuse a treatment, on the basis of relevant information
2. This right confers a duty on healthcare professionals to provide relevant information in a clear and non-coercive manner suited to the patient.

Opinions differ over many related issues. How and when must consent be obtained formally? Must consent be fully informed? How much information is required before consent can be considered informed consent and can we find the middle ground with valid if not fully informed consent?[12] Can one person consent to medical treatment on behalf of another person? The problems abound. What is clear is that the law considers any touching without prior permission to be an assault or battery, and leaves practitioners open to litigation. So why is informed consent so important?

Consider Case 10.

Case 10
The uninformed patient

In August, Hamish Strachan, aged 76, took to his bed. He had been diagnosed with a viral infection a month earlier and vague symptoms had persisted. Finally, his wife Joyce, aged 68, called the GP. The GP couldn't find anything specific wrong, but blood tests showed a haemoglobin of 8. Mr Strachan was referred to a geriatrician and admitted for a blood transfusion. He was discharged feeling dramatically better. During admission, prostatic surface antigen (PSA) results indicated metastatic prostatic cancer. The GP received a discharge note informing him that the patient had returned home and was prescribed steroid tablets. Arrangements were also made for the district nurse to provide Mr Strachan with monthly hormone injections of Zoladex.

On the surface, this case doesn't seem very remarkable. A patient sought help and received it. In similar circumstances the carers, including the patient's wife, could not be faulted for their behaviour and no concerns arise about whether the patient's autonomy has been respected or compromised.

However, a later development reported by the GP does raise some cause for concern.

Case 10 continued...
The GP reports

'I dropped in to see Mr Strachan while I was doing my house calls. I had received a discharge note to say that he had been diagnosed with metastatic prostate cancer and that he was now at home and on medication. His wife came out to meet me on the stairs and said "You do know that Hamish has not been told and is not to know". I was taken aback. I'd had no communication from the hospital about this. I assumed this was a decision that she had made.

I went in to see Mr Strachan, who was looking much better and said he felt fine. He asked me nothing about his diagnosis or treatment, even when I asked him how he got on with his transfusion and his new medication. (He is on monthly Zoladex injections and cyproterone as well as steroids.)

I wanted to talk more to Mrs Strachan but there is no privacy in their flat. However, she stopped me outside their door and said that she realized he had to find out some time but not now as he will only worry about her and what she will do without him. She seemed genuinely concerned.

I visited him again 2 weeks later. He said that he was feeling fine, gaining weight – even eating puddings that he never used to bother with before, according to his wife – presumably because of his steroids. She looked strained, but composed as always. In fact, she had already set the table for tea. I'm sure he doesn't know his diagnosis. I tried to give him the opportunity to ask me questions but he seemed genuinely unconcerned.

I never had any word about it from the geriatrician. I feel uncomfortable about this situation. What right does she have to keep this information from him?'

The case raises issues about the importance of informed consent and the degree to which consent needs to be explicit or implicit.

We will look at a variety of concepts related to informed consent, trying always to relate them to his and other cases. We will look at the different levels of consent (informed, voluntary, involuntary, non-voluntary, implied and explicit) and will contrast informed and valid consent. We will also consider the amount of information that a patient might need, the issue of competence, whether the patient standard or the professional standard is adopted, the issue of relevant or harmful information, how information is imparted and the practitioner's responsibilities for this, the issue of consent for research and, finally, proxy consent.

The value of informed consent
The law takes a very serious view of informed consent and requires consent for any medical procedure.[8] Without prior consent, touching, no matter how well intentioned, is considered an assault and can be treated as negligence, malpractice and, in extreme situations, is punishable as a criminal act of violence. The reason for this is founded on the principle of bodily integrity. All persons are considered to have the right to control over their own bodies. Human rights conventions, such as those endorsed by the United Nations[9] and, more recently, the Human Rights Act 1998 in the UK, include related articles in defence of the individual's liberty of person and freedom from unnecessary coercion, freedom from torture and of self-determination. All of these recognize the value of individual autonomy as it relates to the liberty of the person to be self-determining and to maintain control over what happens to the individual's own body. The requirement for informed consent helps protect this.

Furthermore, seeking informed consent is a means of respecting individual autonomy in the patient. It gives patients an opportunity to consider the information relevant to their own case, to deliberate upon it and reach a decision that reflects their own values and wishes. The upshot of this is that it maintains trust in the healing relationship, an essential ingredient to cooperation, candour and success.

In the case described, Mr Strachan is unable to give full informed consent because he does not have the information required to do so; namely he has not been told that he has cancer. He will not be able to give his consent in an informed manner, nor will he be able to make important decisions about the management of his own care. Does he want therapy for his cancer? How much intervention is he willing to accept? Has he made his final arrangements, fulfilled his life goals and said his last goodbyes? When the time comes, does he want to die at home or in hospice? Mr Strachan will be unable to answer any of these questions because he has not been informed of his illness and prognosis. The control of his case is no longer in his hands. Later on, if he discovers the truth about the conspiracy of silence that prevented him from making these important decisions, he could become angry and distrustful of the care-providers, including his wife. Clear harms begin to surface.

All of these provide significant generalizable reasons for protecting the individual's right to give consent or refusal. It demonstrates that informed consent protects personal autonomy, bodily integrity and trust in the practitioner/patient relationship. Practitioners must respect this or they are negligent. The matter is that simple. Or is it?

Consider why it may be unnecessary or impossible to obtain informed consent for treatment.

Voluntary, involuntary, non-voluntary consent[10]
The General Medical Council is among many international medical governing bodies that recognize the need to obviate informed consent in some cases. Chief among these are emergency situations when individuals are unable to consent. This could be because they are unconscious, a minor or not competent to give consent. What can a doctor do in such cases? The options are fairly clear. Ideally, a patient can give voluntary informed consent and be treated according to particular wishes. Where this is impossible, a doctor can do one of three things. First, the doctor could refrain from treating anyone who is not able to give informed consent. This would protect bodily integrity but would also mean that some people would die unnecessarily, or at least suffer serious consequences because their illness or injury went untreated.

The second option is to go ahead and treat anyway. This would ensure lives were always saved and would also limit permanent damage where patients were left untreated until they could give their consent. This is a caring option but it is also paternalistic because it assumes all people wish to be treated, which they might not. To treat someone against his or her express refusal is involuntary treatment and is unlawful and unethical because it violates personal autonomy and bodily integrity. It is on this basis that some people accuse doctors of malpractice when they are resuscitated against their express wishes. It might seem odd on the surface but some sufferers of serious illnesses would prefer to die peacefully than to have their lives extended simply because of a successful resuscitation. This will be discussed further in Chapters 5 and 6.

So where does this leave the doctor? The third choice offers a middle ground concerning informed consent and offers guidance for practitioners who wish to help but are not able to gain informed consent beforehand. This third option permits the healthcare practitioner to perform as much as necessary to stabilize the patient to such an extent as it permits competent informed consent.

A doctor is justified by necessity in proceeding without the patient's consent if a condition is discovered in an unconscious patient for which treatment is necessary in the sense that it would be, in the circumstances, unreasonable to postpone the operation to a later date. Postponement of treatment is, however, to be preferred if it is possible to wait until the patient is in a position to give consent.[11]

Treating in this situation would be termed non-voluntary because it is neither voluntary (in that it is not performed with patient knowledge or request) nor involuntary (because it is not performed in direct opposition to patient wishes). Instead, it is performed without the patient having any true understanding of the procedure but on the assumption that most reasonable people would voluntarily consent to this type of emergency care.

That makes things fairly clear for emergency situations where patients are incapable of giving voluntary informed consent. However, Mr Strachan was neither in an emergency situation, in that his death was not imminent, nor did he appear to be incapable of giving consent. This raises a further distinction in the idea of consent.

Implied versus explicit consent
Although Mr Strachan was unable to give informed consent because he was unaware of the information regarding his true condition, he arguably gave some kind of consent. He permitted the healthcare professionals involved in his case to provide him with care without refusing or questioning what they did. His unquestioning acquiescence gave the care team an understanding that they had permission to proceed. This is a form of implied consent. Never fully verbalized, certainly not written and signed, it nevertheless appeared to be consistent with Mr Strachan's wishes. Is that enough?

Ordinarily, formal explicit consent is preferred over implied consent. This protects patients by providing them with an opportunity to comprehend the illness and recommended treatment. It permits patients to question and learn about risks and options that may be available. It also protects the healthcare providers because it ensures that patients have actually given permission for the treatment to proceed. Without this there is ambiguity and coincidence at best. At worst, the upshot can be disagreement, loss of trust and accusations of malpractice.

Consent to consultation is implied to a certain extent when patients come to see a doctor, i.e. in the ambulatory setting. This is not necessarily the case with inpatients, who should be asked if they are agreeable to being interrogated and examined. Use of a chaperone or a third party at history taking and physical examination is a desirable moderator of medical consultations. The chaperone can serve to support the patient and the professional, both of whose interests are thereby safeguarded: the patient against abuse, verbal or physical; the professional against misunderstanding or malicious allegations.

There are situations where implied consent is sufficient. For instance, it is unnecessary to seek consent for the minutiae of treatment. Thus, once a patient has given explicit permission for a surgical treatment to proceed, it is acceptable to assume that the consent includes preoperative procedures such as pulse and blood pressure readings. No formal consent would be required for these because they are considered necessary, inclusive parts of the procedure. Nevertheless, patient autonomy and dignity are still involved, so offering explanations of what is about to be done and why, and then waiting for some sign of acquiescence, is not merely polite but helps to preserve the patient's dignity, which will also maintain trust.

Formal consent ought to be made as a written document and, ideally, patients should be given sufficient time to consider and discuss the information they have been given. In rare situations where this is not possible, verbal consent can be sufficient provided it is witnessed and the patient is again adequately informed. Informal consent need only be verbal.

Informed versus valid consent[12]

Mr Strachan's consent will have been more or less implied to the extent that he had no knowledge of his condition or treatment, but accepted whatever was done to him without any request for information. Even so, the team members attached to his case reportedly expressed their unease over treating someone who was unaware of his illness.

Consider why this would be the case:

- List reasons in favour of informing individuals about the details of their case

- List reasons against informing individuals about the details of their case

---

To make a decision on little information might appear to be irresponsible, especially when current trends in consumer-style medical treatment try to encourage as much patient involvement as possible. It would be plausible to argue that demand for respect of patient autonomy brings with it the reciprocal burden of patient responsibility. If patients want practitioners to respect their choices, they need to make responsible, well-reasoned informed choices, not merely comply with the suggestions and requests of doctors. In this view, Mr Strachan is acting irresponsibly by not seeking to know more about his care, which calls his consent into question.

Taken a different way, however, Mr Strachan has the right to know or not to know as he chooses. This need not call his ability to make choices into question. Rather, he ought to be permitted to give his consent on the basis of what he chooses to know, namely that he trusts and respects his carers enough to comply with their suggested course of action. Thus Mr Strachan can be said to have given valid, rather than informed consent, as his cognitive abilities and reasoning skills are not under question and he can be described as competent. He is not fully informed but this is irrelevant to his ability to act competently and make a choice to give his consent.

The advantage of requiring valid consent instead of informed consent is that valid consent does not require the patient to have all information relevant to his or her case. Although there are strong reasons for a person having all relevant information before making a decision, especially an important decision, there are also significant reasons against this. Chief among the reasons in favour is that it would interfere with an individual's ability to make a balanced decision if they were limited to the amount of available information. However, no one can be fully informed, for example of consequences of a chosen action. This would require clairvoyance about future events and knowledge of unforeseen circumstances. As we are not graced with the ability to know the future, most of us act in an uninformed way, to some extent, all the time.

Information – how much is enough?

Patients can be said to have a right to any information they require to make a reasoned decision about their health and healthcare. In circumstances where patients are competent and no harm to third parties will occur from their having such information, it is without question that they deserve to have this knowledge for reasons of autonomy, dignity and trust already explained in this section. The healthcare practitioner's duty of care requires disclosure so that patients can make decisions on the basis of relevant information. To be without relevant information could affect the way the decision is made and will sway the outcome one way or another. If this is the case, the decision could not be said to be wholly voluntary, because it is affected by the limited way in which the patient perceives the situation.[13]

The quantity of information is problematic in another way. Most patients are not professionally trained healthcare providers. When we are patients, we seek professional care because we lack the knowledge and information and professional distance to heal ourselves. Those we approach for assistance have had years of training and experience to enable them to make reasoned decisions and often appropriate diagnoses and treatment. It would be almost impossible to duplicate all the knowledge and information available to the professional, and to do so would be overwhelming. Thus it is necessary to filter and clarify the relevant information to ensure its quantity and complexity does not overwhelm the patient.

Competence

As we have seen, there are times when patients are incapable of autonomous or rational thought and it is therefore inappropriate to expect them to understand information or to make decisions based upon it. Competence or mental capacity will therefore play a significant role in informed consent.

But how competent do people need to be to be able to make appropriate decisions? For that matter, how informed must they be? It goes without saying that not everyone is fully rational or competent enough to give

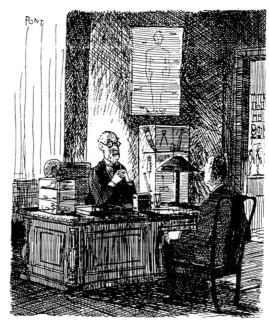

'We must on no account permit anyone to give us a shock, Mr. Pembridge. The least shock of any sort would in our present state of health be sure to kill us immediately.'

Figure 3.1
It is necessary to ensure that information does not overwhelm the patient. (Reproduced with permission of Punch Ltd.)

fully informed consent. This would require being in a position to deliberate upon all information relevant to make the decision, which in most cases would include an overwhelming amount of information. In Chapter 2 (p. 24–26), we addressed consent for non-competent individuals, namely, minors and unconscious people or people with intellectual disabilities. Here, we consider the notion of degrees of competence. In our case study, Mr Strachan presents as if he were competent. Certainly, no mention is made of a possible loss of ability to reason or make decisions. He is 76 but has given no indication of cognitive impairment or dementia. Thus, Mr Strachan is competent and should be in a position to give informed consent. So why is he not asking for information to do so? Perhaps it is because he has sufficient trust in his doctors, nurses and wife to undergo what they recommend without question. Most people might prefer to have more information but he is satisfied with what he does have and unquestioningly accepts his fate. Should he be permitted to do this? It is in keeping with the principle of autonomy that he is free to accept or reject what he wishes. Thus, his acceptance, however subtle, is implied by his compliance. This makes the act of providing him with care lawful, and even ethical, because it is respectful of his choice not to know. Now, suppose Mr Strachan was mildly delirious or suffering from mild dementia. Would he still be able to give consent? In some cases the response to this is no, because the cognitive impairment involved would restrict his ability to make reasoned decisions. But in other ways it could be that Mr Strachan is capable of making choices for himself. A person might be unable to make decisions about money and still be able to express a level of pain and consent to receiving treatment for it.

To answer our questions, then, provided individuals demonstrate a sufficient degree of competence, they are free to make a choice based on whatever amount of information they wish to have – even if this is very little.

The patient standard or the professional standard?
The issue of how much information and what information is relevant is still being debated. Different legal systems have different approaches. In the UK, the professional standard seems to be favoured, while the US and Australia have adopted a patient standard:

> Given a patient standard, the quality of information will be judged from the viewpoint of the prudent – or the particular – patient; under the professional standard, it will be that of the prudent doctor.[14]

The professional standard requires the divulging of information the doctor, or a reasonable body of professional opinion, sees as relevant or useful for the patient. This

protects therapeutic privilege because it permits the doctor 'to withhold information which would merely serve to distress or confuse the patient'.[15]

The problem with this is that the balance of power is placed on the side of the healthcare professionals, who decide what information is worth disclosing and what ought to be withheld. This is a paternalistic position in that it is intended to protect patients from harm. But, like most paternalistic behaviour, it limits patient autonomy and is founded on an implication that the doctor can know better than the patient what is in the patient's best interest; a belief that is counterintuitive when it is applied to autonomous adults.

It is for this reason that the patient standard has been adopted in some countries. The justification for this is that people make decisions for reasons that go beyond pure clinical information. We make decisions based on social relationships, work commitments and personal preferences and experiences. For example, patients who are Jehovah's Witnesses will make healthcare decisions based on their religious commitments and not just on the basis of clinical information. It is natural that healthcare professionals, no matter how experienced they may be, will have only limited knowledge of the individual patient before them. Thus doctors and nurses can reasonably be expected to make valid clinical decisions but ought not to be expected to know how these will impact of the whole of a person's life. For this reason, namely the limitations of human knowledge, it is best for individuals to decide for themselves what is relevant information for making a reasoned decision. The chief counterargument to this brings us back full circle to the therapeutic privilege and the importance of protecting patients from harmful information.

Relevant or harmful information?
What information is pertinent and what is not is difficult to determine. Equally difficult is recognizing how much information a

patient requires before it becomes alarmist or disturbing. For example, it can cause great concern to a person about to undergo a procedure that in one out of every 1000 such procedures the patient dies. Is it reasonable for the patient to be told this in advance? What if the chances of death are 1 in 10 000? 1 in 10 000 000? We can argue that information needs to be disclosed, but at what point does the disclosure become irrelevant, or worse, harmful?

The notion of the Bolam principle will be discussed in depth in Chapter 4; here, we raise it as a possible cut-off point for disclosure. The Bolam test, as it is called, echoes the professional standard of disclosure by stating that 'a doctor is not negligent if he acts in accordance with a practice accepted at the time as proper by a responsible body of medical opinion'.[16] Thus, where information-sharing is concerned, doctors can divulge whatever they think is reasonable and will not be faulted for this if it can be proved that other doctors would have done the same in similar circumstances. This leaves a high degree of freedom for doctors to decide what is relevant and what is not, which is justifiable because it acknowledges the professional's expertise and authority. On the other hand, it might not be satisfactory to many for the prime reason that doctors, as fallible human beings, can make mistakes in their estimation of the relevance of information to a particular person. After all, it is the particular person who will be affected by the outcome of the choice and not the doctor, and why shouldn't patients who have to live with the outcome decide what is relevant and what is not? In addition, patients will include other factors in their decision making beyond purely clinical ones and, for this reason, need to be permitted to view all options in their own contextual light before giving their consent to any one. In this view, the reasonable doctor's perspective would be replaced by that of the reasonable patient. Which brings us back to the problem of the potential harm information can cause to the decision-making process.

One reason against full disclosure that crops up fairly often is when information might be psychologically damaging, such as diagnoses of psychiatric illness. Not all patients with psychiatric illnesses are incompetent to make balanced decisions on the basis of relevant information; an irrational decision is not necessarily an incompetent decision.[17] A decision we perceive to be irrational might simply be one with which we disagree. Patients ought to be supported to make even bizarre choices for themselves provided these do not interfere to a great extent with other people's freedoms. This should be protected unless a flaw in their reasoning can be detected.[18] Thus, at least some psychiatric patients will be capable of giving informed consent. However, they might not be given enough information to allow them to make an informed decision. Some psychiatrists argue that telling patients they are delusional, for example, can interfere with the trust between doctor and patients and prevent patients from seeking valuable help. In such cases, patients could be given an opportunity to consent to treatment or even refuse it, but their decision will be based on limited information.[19] Once again, we have an example of consent that is valid without being informed.

How information is imparted
The way information is imparted to patients will help resolve the issue of harmful information and help to ensure the voluntariness of the decision. Good communication skills can help doctors impart the information in ways that are less disturbing or confusing for patients. For this reason, students of healthcare professions will be required to take communication skills classes and practise their skills with one another or with simulated patients.[20]

It is probably impossible to determine the optimal elements for consent, especially in the medical context where the complexity of the information and emotional states of the patient and family interfere with comprehension and decision-making. Nevertheless, it is incumbent upon healthcare professionals to try their best to ensure maximum understanding and voluntariness. The following case illustrates how important this can be.

Case 11
Retention of organs at post-mortem

In the late 1990s, information surfaced about the retention of organs at post-mortem without prior consent. The story was especially poignant because it involved the retention of child and infant organs without parental knowledge. Parents who discovered that their children's organs had been retained felt betrayed and violated.

Although patients' groups and relatives condemned the arrogance of the medical profession, Professor John Lilleyman, president of the Royal College of Pathologists, apologized on behalf of his college. He maintained that 'there was never any perverse or devious intent' behind the way pathologists around the country behaved, and he insisted that organs were retained for educational purposes.[21] Mostly, this was to facilitate research into the conditions that caused the children's deaths, to help discover cures and diagnostic tests to prevent similar tragedies for future families.

The UK's Chief Medical Officer, Professor Liam Donaldson, was quoted as saying of these practices:

They belong to an era where decisions were made for patients, not with them. We must ensure that clinical care for future patients is improved through good post-mortem practice. But what is important is that the rights of individuals are respected and that consent is properly obtained. We need to put in place a robust modern system to do this.[22]

What concerns us most in this case is the possibility that lack of information so undermined the trust among those directly involved that it engendered a culture of mistrust in the wider public. Images of bizarre collections of jarred hearts, brains and livers stored in dark laboratories for decades began to haunt us.

After the discovery, review groups called for stricter codes of practice on the matter, especially where informed consent was concerned.[23] They described as essential to valid consent several elements relevant to disclosure:

- The person who imparts the information should be of appropriate status, as some patients accept information more readily if it is provided with authority. This might seem good but can intimidate the patient into not asking questions or accepting what they ordinarily would reject. Thus it can be a form of coercion
- The level and clarity of information must be suitable for the patient's individual level of comprehension
- The timing of the information will impact on the degree to which the patient will be able to absorb it. For example, it might not be helpful to begin describing all the treatment alternatives to a patient who has just been given a diagnosis of cancer
- How the information is imparted will also impact on the patient's choice. Doctors ought to avoid subtle or overt manipulation of the information to make one option seem more appealing than another.

To best protect patient freedom, it is most desirable if patients can be given time to consider information and be invited to ask questions to clarify. It is also desirable to invite continuous consent, repeating the informal consent procedure throughout the intervention or treatment to permit the patient to withdraw consent at any time. This is especially relevant in the research context, which will be discussed in Chapter 7. In the research setting, the option for participants to withdraw at any time needs to be reiterated. Fears that withdrawal might be refused, will alienate patient from doctor, or spoil the project, need to be allayed.

Proxy consent

Sometimes it is clear that patients are unable to give consent, either because they are unconscious or are minors or incompetent adults. In such cases, some countries permit proxy consent to be given either by a relative or by someone appointed by court authority to do so.

In the case of unconscious or incompetent adults, a proxy decision-maker would need to be found. In England, Wales and Northern Ireland, (and, up until recently, Scotland where new legislation[24] embodies most of the principles and values discussed here, but gives them force of law in the way the rest of the UK does not), the law did not permit a family member to give informed consent on behalf of an adult unless a court had appointed the proxy. Thus, informal requests by doctors for consent to be provided by the spouse of a patient who was already under anaesthetic or considered incompetent due to dementia, for example, were unlawful. Mrs Strachan's decision to withhold information from her husband would have been determined to be unlawful here too, mostly because he was competent to decide for himself but also because she did not have court authority to do so. Despite the legal position on proxies, doctors usually do include family members in decisions when patients are incompetent or unconscious. The reason for this is more than just one of respect for the family. The reason is based primarily on the assumption that the family member will have: (i) knowledge of the patient's values and preferences; and (ii) the best interests of the patient at heart. Of course, this might not necessarily be the case, but in principle the medical professional should be able to rely on those close to patients to supplement information. The only real drawback is that this entails a breach of confidentiality without patient consent.

The issue is even more complicated in the case of minors. Minors can be called incompetent for many purposes. However, it is broadly acknowledged that some children can make reasoned decisions on their own behalf. The law in the UK famously recognizes this possibility with the statutory Gillick test, discussed in greater detail in Chapter 2 (p. 25–26). The Gillick test states that children can consent if they are considered to have 'sufficient understanding and intelligence [to] make up her own mind regarding the matter',[25] and able to consider the physical and emotional aspects of their decision. This eliminates the need for arbitrary cut-off ages that may overlook the needs of sensitive and mature minors.

Otherwise, in most cases, parents have recognized authority to make decisions on behalf of their child. These parental rights stem from parental duty to protect the child's person and property and therefore their rights extend only as far as they protect the interests of the child. Actions that go beyond the child's best interest can be challenged. Thus, for example, a parent can have the right to sterilize an incompetent female child to protect her from pregnancies where it is especially dangerous for her to undergo them. However, it can never be in the interest of a boy to be sterilized because the interests protected by this will be those of the women he might impregnate, and not his own. Therefore, parental authority to sterilize boys is not recognized. It has been recognized where girls are concerned, but not without court approval. This issue is discussed in greater detail in Chapter 8 (p. 142 and 143). Here, it is relevant to reveal how proxy consent must be limited to procedures with demonstrable therapeutic advantages to the child concerned.

Problems of consent

There are several problems associated with informed consent. These include:

- the limits of consent when harm occurs
- consent or refusal to help another person
- consent or refusal to life-saving intervention
- cost and utilitarian critiques of consent.

The law in most cases easily handles the first of these. It concerns the possibility that people can defend a harmful or illegal act on the grounds that they had consent from the person harmed. Hence, thieves cannot use as their defence the fact that victims agreed to hand over their wallet rather than be shot. Likewise, 'consent will not normally render legitimate a serious physical injury'.[26] This is especially relevant in considering the risks of treatment or research. A person ought not to be asked to consent to any risks unless they are justifiable in light of that person's ability to benefit from whatever risky treatment they will undergo. This is considered under the distinction of therapeutic and non-therapeutic treatment. Where patients stand to gain from the treatment, say chemotherapy for cancer, they might choose to weigh the possible risks against the likelihood of benefit and decide accordingly. Where the intervention will have no therapeutic benefit to the individual, that person ought to be protected from being asked to take the risks involved. For example, a person whose imminent death will not be decelerated by experimental treatment should not be required to take-on risks or hazards such as nausea or other discomfort. In such situations, prior consent will not justify the harm incurred.

The second problem associated with consent is more complicated. What happens when people refuse to give their consent to help another person? The protection of bodily integrity will generally allow for this. No one can be forced to undergo any treatment without giving permission. This will include the right of an individual to refuse to give blood samples for police investigation or even to refuse to donate a life-saving organ. Many would condemn these choices but courts have repeatedly justified the right of the individual to refuse to help others in this way by appeal to the right of bodily integrity. We might give moral disapproval to the choice but cannot force people to undergo a violation to their person, even if doing so will help save the life of another person.

The third problem with informed consent comes when patients refuse to consent to life-saving or other significant intervention. This is classically encountered when a patient who is a Jehovah's Witness refuses a life-saving blood transfusion.[27] The doctor, ideally, should be prepared for this, and recognize refusal to cooperate or participate as the right of the patient, despite this seeming to make evaluation incomplete, and even to waste time. The best interests of the patient might be served by the transfusion being performed and, in such a situation, it is totally ethical for the doctor to try to persuade the patient of this. Rarely, with competent patients, is it either necessary or acceptable to overrule patient wishes. Two possible examples in cancer care, where uncomfortable investigations could be life-saving, are sigmoidoscopy for patients with rectal bleeding and mammography for women with a positive family history of breast cancer who present with a blood-stained nipple discharge. 'Therapeutic discretion', where incomplete disclosure of information is used to try to ensure that patients acquiesce is both illegal and negligent, as well as being obviously immoral by virtue of being dishonest (economical with truth).

A fourth and final argument against informed consent is that it is costly. Costly in terms of time and effort it requires for the information to be imparted and understood, and costly in terms of permitting patients to make choices that might not be beneficial in the wider scheme of things. We have already seen how patients might refuse a life-saving treatment that, on balance, it would be in their own best interest to accept. In addition to this, patients could also choose to refuse a treatment, or they might prefer a treatment that has costs for others as well. We respect autonomy when we respect a parent's decision not to vaccinate his or her child against the measles. However, this could put the child in danger of developing the measles and the potentially devastating side-effects. Moreover, it places other children who are too young to have the vaccine at risk of catching the measles from the first child. A utilitarian reaction to this would be to restrict the choice of the parent and justify it by the maximization principle, saying it is in the interests of the greater number of potential measles sufferers if all children are vaccinated. Utilitarianism might acknowledge the violation of individual liberties this involves but still consider the restriction justified for the good of the many. A similar justification can be used to explain the actions of the pathologists involved in the organ retention case. Once again, the potential benefits to the population at large were deemed sufficient justification for intruding on the autonomy of the few. The position calls to the fore this moving deontological response made in 1967 by research doctor MH Pappworth:

> No physician is justified in placing science or the public welfare first and his obligation to the individual, who is his patient or subject, second. No doctor, however great his capacity or original his ideas, has the right to choose martyrs for science or for the general good.[28]

Summary

One of the classic legal cases regarding informed consent is that of *Sidaway* v. *Board of Governors of the Bethlem Royal Hospital and the Maudsley Hospital*. In the appeal to the initial findings, the Justice (Sir John Donaldson) expressed concern that 'the definition of the duty of care was a matter for the law which could not stand by if the profession, by an excess of paternalism, denied their patients a real choice'.[29] The right to give consent protects patients' freedom to choose.

Rights of practitioners

As the dominant motivation for practising medicine is both beneficent and non-

maleficent, medical practitioners have a right not to be exploited commercially either by their employers or by patients. Employing authorities should not create excessive demands and medical seniors ought not to exploit junior and trainee practitioners with expectations of extremely long hours, e.g. when colleagues are sick or when waiting lists are increasing.

Doctors have the right to decline to respond to excessive demands by attention-seeking, histrionic patients, e.g. an elderly, socially isolated patient or individuals with chronic non-life-threatening conditions, e.g. a woman with a recurrent non-puerperal breast abscess.

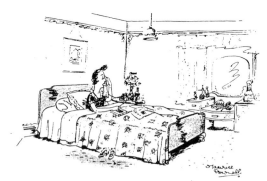

'And on your way here, Doctor, would you mind calling at the fishmonger's?'

Figure 3.2
Patients can make excessive demands. (Reproduced with permission of Punch Ltd.)

Doctors have rights in relation to criticism and complaints. They can expect that any such will be made initially in a private setting, rather than in front of other people, such as on a ward round or in a consulting room. Ideally, the manner in which a criticism is made should be such that the professionals whose performance is being criticized should be encouraged to review their own performance in the matter to detect any errors or under-performance. Where such insight cannot be inculcated, the criticism should be given in a non-confrontational way without aggression. Where a formal complaint has to be delivered to a doctor, that individual is entitled to have another individual present as both a witness and potentially as an advocate. Formal complaints should be in writing, preferably with the identity of the complainant stated. Recognized complaints procedures for both general practitioners and hospital doctors exist (see Chapter 4).

Doctors have the right (as well as the responsibility) to continued professional development and life-long learning. A corollary is that they are entitled to paid study leave, except in exceptional circumstances. This means that employing authorities, except in circumstances of exceptional demands being made on the services they provide, should allow time and money for their medical employees to continue their professional learning.

Finally, doctors have the right not to have to continue to treat patients with whom they feel incompatible. Safeguards for the patients must exist in this situation. Usually, the withdrawing doctor has the responsibility of identifying another colleague who will provide continued care for that patient.

Like many person-to-person human interactions, doctor–patient relationships don't always work well. There is always the possibility that the doctor might not 'like' the patient, and vice versa. As stated above, doctors have the right to decline to continue to see particular patients, subject to the caveat that the health of the patients will not suffer and that the declining doctor ensures that other practitioners will take on responsibility of providing care for those patients.

An issue that is close to this, but not quite so extreme, is that of patients whose doctors come to dread having to consult with or visit them. Such patients are sometimes labelled 'heart-sink patients'.

> Is it desirable, ethical and helpful to label patients in this way?

Case 12
The heart-sink patient

Maurice is a 70-year-old man who returned to live in the UK from overseas 5 years ago. Since his return, he has complained repeatedly that he is suffering from abdominal pain. This pain causes him considerable discomfort. He maintains a good weight. Indeed, he is somewhat overweight, and also complains of constipation. Maurice has been extensively and repeatedly investigated but no cause for his pain has been found. He lives with his wife who is concerned about, as well as patient with him. She thinks he drinks too much beer, which she believes worsens his symptoms. Frequently, Maurice seems to be depressed. When offered consultations with a clinical psychologist and a psychiatrist, he refuses. He insists on taking pain killers of a type that are known to cause constipation. He is reluctant to leave his house, to take exercise or to participate in any activity except going to his local pub.

When Maurice sees his general practitioner, or when he is at hospital clinics, most of the healthcare professionals whisper to each other 'Oh, Maurice is here again! Who is going to see him today?' in other words, Maurice has a reputation as a heart-sink patient.

Clearly, in approaching any patient, doctors must put the welfare of that patient first. Frequently, this necessitates doctors making sacrifices of their own patience and time. When the patient acquires a label, there is a great risk that doctors will be less willing to give of their patience and time. Other members of the healthcare team will make similar assumptions based on the label, and this can cause them to alter their behaviour in prejudicial ways. Thereby, the patient may be disadvantaged – even done harm.

> How can 'labelling' patients do them harm?

For Maurice, the fact that he has become labelled means that his doctor's mind might be closed to the possibility that there is an unconsidered, even remediable cause for his persistent symptoms. Maurice himself, each time he comes to clinic or surgery, is likely to sense the unwelcoming reception given to him. This could make him reluctant to relax and to speak spontaneously and easily about what is happening in his life. So opportunities can be lost for his doctor to learn about medically important features of his condition.

During the consultation, the fact that Maurice has been 'labelled' could result in him being given a more cursory physical examination than he would otherwise have had, so newly appearing physical signs might be missed. At the end of the consultation, his doctor might be content to let Maurice continue with his preferred medication, instead of spending time to persuade him to try a potentially more helpful alternative. Finally, when decisions for follow-up appointments are made, Maurice, and other heart-sink patients, will be given as long an interval as possible, because of the dread of having to try to deal with him again.

The other alternative for Maurice is that his best interests are served by his being told that, despite his persistent symptoms, his doctors, having investigated him as carefully as they know how (which might have included a second opinion), cannot find nything wrong with him. They would encourage him to regard himself as fit, and not arrange any further follow-up appointment.

Despite our tendency as human beings to stereotype, it is preferable professionally for doctors not to 'label' patients and to avoid adopting tags that are designated by others to those who seek advice from us.

Rights of society

The rights of society will be discussed in greater detail in Chapter 9. Here, it is relevant to raise one salient point. As, in many societies, the costs and opportunities for doctors to acquire their professional training comes from the society itself, that society has the right to expect the doctors it has trained to serve the society by way of appreciation and repayment. Equitable arrangements for this vary, but should be capable of being achieved with mutual agreement.

Conclusion

This chapter covers a diversity of important issues, each of which could have filled a book on its own. It is worth reviewing what has been discussed because the focus on the relationship between patients and their practitioners will reflect on all future chapters in this text.

So far, we have looked at the following aspects of the doctor–patient relationship, which are designed to protect patients as well as practitioners and ensure the best possible patient care:

- rights of patients, practitioners and society
- consent
- patient competence
- confidentiality and exceptions
- difficult patients.

There are many more issues to be looked at in relation to these. In the following chapters we will consider specific issues and general theories that will help elucidate what has been discussed so far. We hope to help draw conclusions about the best way to provide excellent and essential care as you are being trained to provide it.

Notes and references

1 Downie RS. The ethics of medical involvement in torture. J Medical Ethics 1993; 19:135–137.

2 General Medical Council. Duties of a doctor: Confidentiality. London; GMC: 1995:2.

3 *Tarasoff* v. *Regents of the University of California* (1976) 551 P 2d 334

4 Walzer Leavitt J. Typhoid Mary: captive to the public's health. Boston, MA: Beacon Press; 1996.

5 Brazier M. Medicine, patients and the law. Middlesex: Penguin Books; 1992:58.

6 For a detailed list of appropriate disclosure of patient information, see the Caldicott Committee Report on the Review of Patient-identifiable Information produced for the NHS Executive in December 1997. Available: http://www.doh.gov.uk/confiden/crep.htm

7 Recently, the Caldicott Report has covered many of these considerations in British policy.

8 As expressed in *Schloendorff* v. *Society of New York Hospital* 105 NE 92 (NY 1914). In the UK, see A-G's reference (No 6 of 1980) [1981] QB 715, [1981] 2 All ER 1057.

9 The United Nations Universal Declaration of Human Rights. Available: http://www.un.org/Overview/rights.html

10 Mason J, McCall Smith R. Law and medical ethics. 5th edn. London: Butterworths; 1999:246.

11 Mason J, McCall Smith R. Law and medical ethics. 5th edn. London: Butterworths; 1999:247.

12 Syse A. Norway: valid (as opposed to informed) consent. The Lancet 2000; 356:1347–1348.

13 *Sidaway* v. *Board of Governors of the Bethlem Royal Hospital and the Maudsley Hospital* [1985] AC 871.

14 Mason J, McCall Smith R. Law and medical ethics. 5th edn. London: Butterworths; 1999:279.

15 Mason J, McCall Smith R. Law and medical ethics. 5th edn. London: Butterworths; 1999:279.

16 Mason J, McCall Smith R. Law and medical ethics. 5th edn. London: Butterworths; 1999:280.

17 Draper H. Anorexia nervosa and respecting a refusal of life-prolonging therapy: a limited justification. Bioethics 2000; 14(2):120–133.

18 Brown J et al. Challenges in caring: explorations in nursing and ethics. London: Chapman & Hall; 1992:65.

19 McLean S, Manson S. A patient's right to know: information disclosure, the doctor and the law. Aldershot: Dartmouth; 1989:85.

20 See, for example, Lloyd M, Bor R. Communication skills for medicine. Edinburgh: Churchill Livingstone; 1996.

21 Abbasi K Summit signals a change in the law on organ retention. Br Med J 2001; 322:125.

22 Abbasi K Summit signals a change in the law on organ retention. Br Med J 2001; 322:125.

23 Royal College of Pathologists. Guidelines for the retention of tissues and organs at post-mortem (2000). Review Group on Retention of Organs at Post-mortem. Available: http://www.show.scot.nhs.uk/scotorgrev

24 Adults with Incapacities Act Scotland, 2000. Available at: http://www.scotland-legislation. hmso.gov.uk/legislation/scotland/acts 2000/20000004.

25 Brazier M. Medicine, patients and the law. Middlesex: Penguin Books; 1992:329–353.

26 Mason J, McCall Smith R. Law and medical ethics. 5th edn. London: Butterworths; 1999:245.

27 See: Gillon R. Refusal of potentially life-saving blood transfusions by Jehovah's Witnesses: should doctors explain that not all JWs think it's religiously required? J Medical Ethics 2000; 26:299–301 and Elder L. Why some Jehovah's Witnesses accept blood and conscientiously reject official Watchtower Society blood policy. J Medical Ethics 2000; 26:375–380.

28 Pappworth MH. Human guinea pigs. Boston, MA: Beacon Press: 1967:27.

29 As quoted in Mason J, McCall Smith R. Law and medical ethics. 5th edn. London: Butterworths; 1999:281.

4

Accountability

We are all under greater pressure to prove our worth and justify our continued presence in the workplace. Doctors should not be an exception. The very nature of their job demands that they come under open, tough and fair scrutiny.

Editorial in *The Herald*, 6 January 2000

It has been suggested that medicine is much less accountable than other professions that are responsible for the safety and wellbeing of other people. A leading article in *The Times* stated[1]:

After Dr Shipman, after the Bristol heart surgery case, the Ritchie inquiry[2] into the malpractice and incompetence of Rodney Ledward will destroy any public illusions that doctors or health service managers are anywhere near as accountable for their actions, and even their most lethal mistakes, as they should be…the culture of complacency must end.

In the UK, the government is taking steps to promote a culture of clinical excellence by making individuals accountable for setting, maintaining and monitoring standards.[3] The concept of 'clinical governance' has been introduced as a framework for making health organizations accountable for improving the quality of the services they provide. As *The Times* editorial mentioned above concluded, 'the General Medical Council must do far more, in medical schools, to inculcate in junior doctors attitudes of self-criticism, openness and continuous professional development'. Being held to account is now an integral part of being a doctor.

A radical cultural change is taking place in the world of medicine and it is important that

all doctors understand their responsibilities in promoting public confidence in the healthcare system. Trust between patients and doctors is important and has recently been shaken by the scandals mentioned above.[4] Doctors and all those involved in healthcare must be able to give logical and sustainable explanations of why they decided to act in the way they did when carrying out their duties. This chapter looks at the concept of accountability, as it applies to the healthcare professions, and examines the ways in which individual healthcare professionals can be held to account. In view of the rapidly changing environment, consideration is also given to how future systems may evolve. For the sake of presentation, the discussion will concentrate on doctors; however, the same principles apply to all healthcare professionals. The chapter concludes by considering some practical measures individuals can adopt to facilitate the process of accountability.

Case 13
The Bristol Royal Infirmary Inquiry

In the mid-1990s a story broke that was to change the practice of medicine in the UK forever. Serious concerns about the number of children dying or being left brain damaged after cardiac surgery at Bristol Royal Infirmary led to a wave of public outcry. Not only did the General Medical Council discipline three senior doctors but a Public Inquiry was also conducted between October 1998 and July 2001 to inquire into the management of the care of children receiving complex cardiac surgical services at Bristol Royal Infirmary between 1984 and 1995. The inquiry was one of the longest and most expensive ever held. It heard evidence from 577 witnesses and examined the medical records of 1800 children.

The terms of reference of the inquiry included reaching conclusions from these events and making recommendations that could help secure high-quality care across the NHS.[5]

The final report identified various problems both within the paediatric cardiac surgery department of Bristol Royal Infirmary and more widely in the NHS. These included a lack of leadership, poor organization, a lack of standards, lack of teamwork and a 'club culture'. The extensive recommendations included suggestions for ways in which the NHS could promote:

- respect and honesty in the practice of medicine
- a well-led health service
- competent healthcare professionals
- a culture of safety
- improved standards
- shared learning across boundaries
- public involvement through empowerment.

It is likely that this inquiry will have a major influence on the way the medical profession is regulated and on the culture operating in the NHS in the future.

No easy answers in medicine

Medicine is unique in many ways, dealing as it does quite literally with matters of life and death (Fig. 4.1). Even if the gravity of this is recognized, it is and will remain a fallible practice. To expect doctors to never make mistakes, while at the same time acknowledging that 'to err is human', appears to be logically inconsistent. Lord Justice Nourse once said 'Of all sciences medicine is one of the least exact'.[6] Others have suggested that it is overly simplistic to regard medicine simply as a science, suggesting instead that it is a discrete discipline that draws on many others.[7] At any rate, unlike the work of the precision engineer or analytical chemist, exact outcomes can rarely be promised or guaranteed by doctors. Treatments do not always work, outcomes are often less satisfactory than might be desired by the patients or their carers, and patients will

sometimes die despite the best of care. When the unexpected occurs, or when patients or their relatives are dissatisfied, questions will inevitably be asked about why certain decisions were made and why specific actions were taken or not taken. Clinical governance and audit will also require individuals to account for the standards achieved.[8]

Throughout this book, we have been at pains to emphasize that the complex moral and ethical problems encountered by doctors rarely have one 'correct answer'. When considering the sorts of dilemmas discussed in other parts of this book, there is usually more than one way of looking at a situation. This is not as alarming as it sounds and is not to say that problems cannot be meaningfully analysed. Just because there might be more than one best way of proceeding does not mean that any way will do! However, when an outcome falls short of expectations, questions may well be asked about why alternative courses of action were not followed instead (see p. 78).

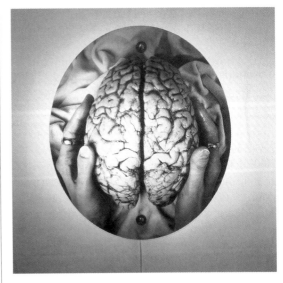

Figure 4.1
The artist's hands cradling a human brain reflect the enormity of the responsibility that comes with caring for the fragile human body. ('Self-portrait' Helen Chadwick 1991 © Helen Chadwick Estate. Reprinted courtesy of the Zelda Cheatle Gallery, London.)

Accountability applies to all facets of a healthcare professional's work, from the practical skill-based components, such as surgical procedures, through the knowledge-based aspects to the more nebulous areas involving attitudes, ethical considerations and judgements. The systems and processes that have developed to scrutinize doctors' decisions are diverse and, as indicated above, are undergoing change. Before looking at them in more depth, it is worth thinking about how we have arrived at the present position and the intellectual framework within which they exist.

Clinical freedom and consumerism

A boy or man wishes to be a doctor. Having learnt as much or as little as he pleases, he can see whatever patients consult him, when it suits him; he can give what advice he pleases, however unorthodox and provide whatever treatment he pleases, however expensive or lethal; he can behave towards his patients however he pleases and extract from them what ever they will pay.[9]

This quotation graphically illustrates some of the issues that need to be considered when discussing clinical freedom and the autonomy of doctors. In fact, the writer – who was arguing that doctors have never been totally free – is perhaps overstating what complete 'clinical freedom' would be like.

- Do you think Sir Theodore Fox's definition of 'old style' clinical freedom is desirable?
- What do you think the practice of medicine would be like if such 'freedom' existed?

In the article from which this extract is taken, the author goes on to state that 'complete freedom is right outside human experience…membership of a profession necessarily involves some additional loss of personal liberty'.

The issue of paternalism in medicine was discussed in Chapter 1 (p. 9), and some authors have attacked the concept of 'clinical freedom' as an undesirable expression of this. So what do doctors mean by clinical freedom, and are there ways of balancing the rights of both doctors and patients to act autonomously? Indeed, is there any reason to assume a conflict between the rights of patients and the rights of doctors? As will be seen, the ways in which doctors are held accountable reflect some of these tensions.

When we think about freedom it is helpful to differentiate the concepts of 'freedom from' and 'freedom to'. In life, we seek freedom from poverty, oppression and imprisonment. Likewise, many advocates of human rights express a desire for people to be free to express themselves, worship as they see fit and associate 'freely' with others.

1. List three things doctors should be free from

2. List three things doctors should be free to do

3. Compare your list with your colleagues'. What would the implications on other parties be if your lists were adopted?

A conflict of interests can arise when one person seeks to exercise his or her freedom to act in a particular way if this action impacts adversely on other people. For example, you might feel that doctors should be free to prescribe whichever drug they wish for their patients. However, if there is a less expensive, less toxic or more effective alternative, how desirable is this freedom? We will consider some of these issues further in the section on resource allocation.

Other examples of where it might be desirable to limit 'clinical freedom' include non-consented examinations and the scope of procedures undertaken during exploratory surgery. There are dangers, however, in going too far in reducing autonomy of doctors. To see the doctor simply as a technician who is under an obligation to provide whatever the client or customer wants or demands undermines the concept we have argued for of joint decision making. Blocking individuals with the acquired expertise to solve problems from using their skills seems to be an illogical use of an expensive resource. Expertise, however, confers power on the individual. How this power is used and responded to by others has been the subject of much debate.[10] To balance the expert power of the doctor, some people have advocated giving more power to patients. The trend towards 'consumerism' and 'consumer empowerment', which emerged in the 1980s, raises questions about how such power can be 'given' to patients, how the use of such powers affects what is offered to patients by their doctors and the health service, and finally how the providers of care are held to account when there is a dispute between them and their patients. This shifting balance of power has given rise to considerable debate and the search for alternative approaches. How did it all start?

When the Welfare State was established in the 1940s, the fledgling NHS was hailed as the flagship of the social reforms. Care was to be offered 'from the cradle to the grave' for all, regardless of the ability to pay. It has been observed that, until the 1970s at least, the established status and prevailing ethos of the medical profession 'created an impenetrable barrier against opinions which challenged medical orthodoxy'.[11] Patients had little power in the early days of the NHS, and rarely sued or complained about their doctors.

Patients, customers or partners?

The ways in which the profession set standards and was held accountable came under scrutiny in the 1980s when the Conservative government of Margaret Thatcher set about reforming the way public services in general, and the NHS in particular, was managed. Exposing the NHS to market forces and competition was part of the government's plan to replace the traditionally professionally based value system of NHS management with a more 'business-like' approach.[12] It was suggested that public services needed to be more responsive to the needs of those who use them. The old image of patients being the passive and grateful recipients of such treatments as their doctors considered right for them was gradually replaced with the concept of consumerism, in which patients became 'customers' who had 'rights' to treatment. This shift, which involved persuading people to think of themselves no longer as patients but as customers, involved proposing significant changes in the relationship and balance of power between doctors and their patients.

It is said that 'the customer is always right' and, certainly, customers who ask shop assistants for goods or services usually expect their demands to be met. Issac-Henry et al.[13] suggest that the term 'customer' is symbolic because it conjures up a view of individuals using services and making choices and, by so doing, influencing the quantity and quality of the services given.

> Do you agree with the suggestion that this applies to users of healthcare?

Other writers have pointed out that customers in the public sector are 'not the same as customers in the market'[14] and that to replace the traditional role of the doctor with that of a supplier of goods and services is highly undesirable.[15] Real people are rarely completely independent and their decision making does not always meet the norms that define rationality. For example, they do not always act in accordance with their own best interests.

More recently, it has been suggested that patients and their doctors should be viewed as partners in a joint venture.[16] Because such a partnership can take different forms, different writers have suggested a range of models that depend upon the clinical context of the encounter between patient and doctor.[17] It has been noted that 'in current healthcare systems, both time and funding constraints can act as disincentives for doctors to explore and respond to patients' preferences regarding the type of partnership they would prefer in the process of making decisions about treatment'.[18]

This change in the relationships within the NHS continues to evolve,[19] but it must be observed that the Conservative government's vision for reforming the Welfare State was never as fully endorsed by the electorate as the founding of the system was 50 years before, in the days after the Second World War. The social changes that have taken place are unlikely to be reversed, however, and, after Mrs Thatcher resigned, her successor introduced the Patient's Charter, which was designed to increase the customer's rights (see Appendix 2). Consumerism within the health service can be seen to encompass a number of important issues, including customer access to information about the service (e.g. hospital league tables),[20] representation and participation in the decision-making process (elected Health Board and Trust directors) and what has been described as 'proper' grievance and redress mechanisms.[21] The concept of consumerism has been criticized on the grounds that it encouraged people to make demands but failed to emphasize reciprocal responsibilities.[22] Traditionally, courts have been reluctant to find that patients who have suffered harm have responsibility for part of their loss, so-called contributory negligence. However, as patients become better informed and command greater levels of autonomy in their treatment, it is possible that judges will expect them to accept more responsibility for their welfare. Already there are signs that some patients' groups are thinking about this issue.[23]

In 1997, a change in government in the UK saw a change in approach and the concept of 'patient partnership' began to be promoted.[24] The issues relating to the extent to which people will want or be able to take an active role in decision making have been explored in Chapter 2, but it is worth noting that the way individuals and society regard its relationship with its doctors and healthcare professionals will affect the approach adopted to holding them accountable. Confusion about this relationship and the distribution of power within this arena can cause misunderstandings and tensions in the accountability process.

Ultimately, it must be for society at large rather than the medical profession to decide what sort of doctors it wants and how healthcare professionals fit into society. Unfortunately, the quality of the debate has not been of the highest standard and it remains a challenge to all those concerned with healthcare to move it forward in a thoughtful and intelligent way. Before turning to look at the current grievance and redress procedures, and how they apply to doctors and healthcare professionals, we will pause briefly to consider some of the underlying premises of their foundation.

The use of words like 'grievance' and 'redress' infer that someone or something must be at fault and that they should be made to pay for mistakes. This gives rise to questions about the natural condition of mankind. In the seventeenth century the English thinker Thomas Hobbes published his landmark book 'Leviathan', in which he presented a view of people required to give up their absolute liberty to a supreme ruler or enforcement agency in order to save themselves from the ever-present danger of violent quarrelling due to competition for scarce resources.[25] This work portrayed people as beings essentially driven by selfish motives who need to be controlled to stop them doing 'bad' things. Not long after Hobbes, the philosopher John Locke discussed similar issues in his work 'Second Treatise of Civil Government'.[26] In Locke's view 'men live together according to reason without a common superior on earth'. He suggested that people are motivated internally to want to do their best and require the freedom and resources to do so.

Clearly, the view of mankind adopted by those seeking to make doctors accountable will influence the sort of system they will design. In addition, the view subscribed to by doctors who are being criticized will affect how they respond when their decisions are called into question.

Unfortunately the assumptions sometimes made when ascribing fault or blame can lead to pressures that are counterproductive to the general good of users of healthcare services, as well as contributing to the widely reported levels of dissatisfaction and feelings of persecution within the profession.[27]

Whose fault is it anyway – the individual's or the system's?

When things go wrong it is possible to blame either those involved or the system within which they work. A choice is made between targeting an individual and an institution. In medicine, the focus has traditionally been directed towards individuals, usually those at the 'coal-face' of providing clinical care, such as junior doctors, nurses and surgeons. Although most would acknowledge that 'to err is human', such an approach will inevitably attribute errors to features of an individual's behaviour, such as forgetfulness, inattention, poor motivation, carelessness or recklessness. As Reason[28] points out, the associated countermeasures are:

> …directed mainly at reducing unwanted variability in human behaviour. These methods include poster campaigns that appeal to people's sense of fear, writing another procedure (or adding to existing ones), disciplinary measures, threat of litigation, retraining, naming, blaming, and shaming.

He goes on to suggest that this approach tends to 'treat errors as moral issues, assuming that bad things happen to bad people'. Individuals who believe that this is so will naturally conclude that, when things go wrong, it must be because of their own inadequacies or wickedness. The implications for their self-esteem are obvious. As Reason points out, from some perspectives this approach has much to commend it. Blaming individuals is emotionally, if not financially, more satisfying than targeting institutions. People are viewed as free agents capable of choosing between safe and unsafe modes of behaviour. If something goes wrong, it seems obvious that an individual (or group of individuals) must have been responsible. Reason goes on to describe an alternative way of viewing errors:

> An alternative approach is to view errors as consequences rather than causes, having their origins not so much in the perversity of human nature as in 'upstream' systemic factors. These

include recurrent error traps in the workplace and the organisational processes that give rise to them. Countermeasures are based on the assumption that though we cannot change the human condition, we can change the conditions under which humans work. A central idea is that of system defences. All hazardous technologies possess barriers and safeguards. When an adverse event occurs, the important issue is not who blundered, but how and why the defences failed.[29]

To learn from errors and near misses is the main way that the delivery of healthcare can be made safer. Meanwhile, we will return to consider the main arenas in which doctors are held to account, and where they are likely to have to explain their actions. As you read this section you should think of how these systems are likely to affect practice.

Complaints

When any of us are unhappy about an item we have bought or a service we have received we usually think about complaining. As we have already noted above, there has been a political move to regard medicine as 'just another service', akin to an airline or department store. Part of this trend can be seen in the emphasis placed on an efficient complaint-handling system as an important aspect of contemporary public services, including the health service. A review committee set up by the Secretary of State for Health reported in 1994 that the procedures then in place were over-complex, bewildering and slow, and concluded that 'complainants can face an uphill struggle when using NHS complaints procedures'.[30] The committee, which consulted widely across the health service and with the private service sector, recommended that a new complaints system should be introduced, based

on the set of general principles in Table 4.1. A streamlined system was duly introduced to the NHS in 1996.

> - When did you last complain about a service you received?
> - Consider what you wanted to achieve and whether you were successful. What do you think the effect was on the person you complained to?
> - Discuss your answers with your colleagues.

The review committee's report emphasized that 'the negative associations of complaints – that they happen when something has gone wrong and result in blame for practitioners and staff – must be overcome'. The current NHS complaints procedure has the epithet 'Listening, Acting, Improving' to reflect the underpinning principles of the system. In essence, patients are encouraged to complain directly to the part of the health service with which they are dissatisfied, and there is an expectation that most complaints can be resolved at local level. It is intended that the system will not only hear patients' complaints about the NHS but will also encourage those who work in the service to look at ways of improving it. Because of the emotional engagement of the parties that give rise to the complaint, this can prove extremely difficult sometimes. It is recognized that

Table 4.1
General principles for a complaint-handling system

- Responsiveness
- Quality enhancement
- Cost effectiveness
- Accessibility
- Impartiality
- Simplicity
- Speed
- Confidentiality
- Accountability

doctors find complaints stressful and experience feelings of depression, indignation and doubts about their clinical competence.[31] Perhaps this is because most healthcare professionals see themselves not merely as the suppliers of services but as professionals who engage emotionally and intellectually with their patients. The new procedure is summarized in Figure 4.2.

Level 1 – Local Resolution

The aim of the complaints procedure is to resolve complaints locally wherever possible. Usually this involves the person complained about responding to the complainant in writing or meeting in person to discuss the complaint. By taking patients' concerns seriously, providing clear explanations, and where appropriate an apology, it is hoped that the system will prove satisfactory for all parties in the majority of cases. The evidence suggests that this is very often so.[32] Sometimes the involvement of a lay conciliator as an 'honest broker' or go-between can

help the process of local resolution and all Trusts now provide these free of charge.

Level 2 – Independent Review

When complaints cannot be resolved at local level complainants can request an independent review of their complaint. All Trusts, as well as Health Boards and Health Authorities, have a complaints convenor who considers these requests and can decline the request, return the complaint to local level for a further attempt at resolution or set up an Independent Review Panel (IRP). There is no automatic right to an independent review and complainants must set out the reasons for their continuing grievance and why they are dissatisfied with local resolution.

An IRP is made up of three lay members and is assisted by two clinical assessors drawn from an appropriate speciality if the complaint concerns clinical matters. The IRP's task is to make inquiries into the issues surrounding the complaint to establish if all or part of the complaint can be upheld. The IRP can also make recommendations about systems and ways of working if it feels there are lessons to be learnt from the issues raised by the complaint. This process seems to work best where shortcomings are not simply attributed to an individual who feels scapegoated, but indicates practical ways of identifying best practice and improving the way care is delivered.

Level 3 – Health Service Commissioner (or Ombudsman)

Sitting above the NHS complaints procedures described above is the Health Service Commissioner, who is also known as the Ombudsman. For the sake of clarity, we will refer to him or her by the latter name. The Ombudsman is a senior civil servant who is completely independent of the NHS and has the role of reporting to Parliament about the running of the service, so that the legislature is aware of problems that exist in the service and possible improvements that should be

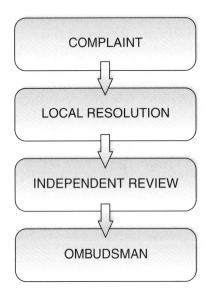

Figure 4.2
An outline of the NHS complaints procedure.

made to it.[33] One way in which the Ombudsman discharges this function is to conduct his or her own inquiries into complaints about poor service and administrative failures. It is up to the Ombudsman which complaints are investigated.

Following such an inquiry, the Ombudsman issues a report setting out his or her findings and conclusions. Every year, the Ombudsman presents a report to Parliament. This usually includes a description of a selection of cases investigated that year, which are felt to raise issues of public interest. Occasionally, doctors and other healthcare workers who have been involved in the complaints are asked to appear before a Select Committee of Parliament to give an account of their actions. This is a very public form of accountability.

The NHS complaints procedure does not (at present) have any provision for offering patients compensation for losses or harm they have suffered. It can be argued that there would be a conflict in doing so whilst at the same time encouraging the open discussion of problems that have arisen. The lack of sanctions in the complaints procedure can, however, leave some complainants dissatisfied. Nor does the complaints system discipline doctors or other healthcare workers. Again, some complainers feel dissatisfied by this situation. In fact, copies of IRP reports are sent to senior managers of the employing or relevant Trust, Authority or Board and it is open to them to initiate disciplinary procedures or refer the matter to a registering body, such as the GMC or UKCC, if they feel such action is appropriate. However, such sanctions are not under the control of the individual who raised the complaint. To recover compensation, individuals need to turn to the civil justice system.

The civil justice system

One of the main purposes of the civil justice system is to provide a mechanism through which individuals can recover monetary compensation for avoidable harm that they have suffered as a result of the 'negligent' acts or omissions of another individual who owed them a duty of care. Cases brought against doctors used to be relatively rare but their number rose steadily during the last two decades of the twentieth century. Figure 4.3 demonstrates the rising trend (noted by the Medical and Dental Defence Union of Scotland) in negligence cases brought against GPs. Some of the reasons behind this trend have been touched on already. In addition, as Dickson[34] observes:

> Along with the rise in the number of claims, there has been a spectacular rise in the sums sued for and awarded. Many patients, who in the past would probably have died following a medical blunder, now, owing to advances in resuscitation, survive. They may, however, be left permanently disabled or even brain damaged and as a consequence need a great deal of help and nursing assistance. This inevitably results in a far larger award than would have been the case if the claim had merely been that of a relative seeking solatium[35] and loss of support.

Negligence is not, of course, a concept related only to the medical profession.

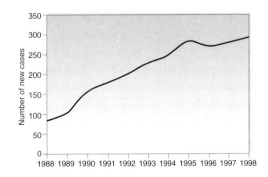

Figure 4.3
The rise of negligence claims against GPs.

Everyone has a duty to avoid harming others. However, it has long been recognized that doctors find the prospect of being accused of being negligent very distressing. Lord Denning once remarked that 'An action for negligence against a doctor is for him unto a dagger. His professional reputation is as dear to him as his body, perhaps more so, and an action for negligence can wound his reputation as severely as a dagger can his body'.[36] Again, this seems to hint that the relationship between doctors and their patients is in some way different from that which exists between other professionals and their clients.

> Do you think Lord Denning's remarks are true today, and if so why?

What is professional negligence?

How do civil courts decide if a doctor has been negligent and a patient should be compensated? Surprisingly, one does not automatically follow the other. The law insists that patients demonstrate that not only was their care suboptimal but also that the doctor's negligence caused them to suffer harm that can be compensated in monetary terms. Many cases against doctors pivot on the vital piece of evidence – 'the causal link'.

Outcomes in clinical medicine can be unpredictable and might not measure up to what either the doctor or patient had hoped for. However, this is not to say that the doctor has been negligent. So how can a standard be set below which a doctor's performance is considered negligent, and how can it be assessed in cases of disagreement?

For the sake of argument, let us suppose that you have asked an architect to design a garage for you. When you commission this architect, you realize that he or she is probably not be the foremost designer in the world, because you probably could not afford to hire such a person. Nor would you expect your

garage to survive rare or unexpected insults such as earthquakes or being run into by a lorry. You could reasonably expect, however, that your architect would at least have the skills to design an ordinary building that could withstand the ordinary stresses such a building could reasonably be expected to be exposed to.

You will see that we have introduced terms such as 'ordinary' and 'reasonable', and these terms are important when thinking about the standard of care required of a doctor. Let us pause briefly to consider a real example that arose in Scotland.

Case 14
Hunter v. Hanley – a case study in medical negligence[37]

Mrs Hunter suffered from a chest infection and was treated by her GP, Dr Hanley, with a course of intramuscular antibiotic injections. During one such injection into her buttock the needle broke and could not be retrieved. Mrs Hunter sued the doctor for his alleged failure to use a suitably heavy gauge hypodermic needle. In court, experts gave evidence that established that if a heavier gauge needle had been used it would have been unlikely to have broken. However, a number of other expert general practitioners gave evidence that at the time in question they would have used the same type of needle as Dr Hanley. His choice of needle was therefore in keeping with the ordinary practice of the time.

Lord President Clyde stated:

> In the realm of diagnosis and treatment there is ample scope for genuine differences of opinion and one man is clearly not negligent merely because his conclusion differs from that of other professional men, nor because he has displayed less skill and knowledge than others would have shown. The true test in establishing negligence in diagnosis or treatment is whether he has been proved to be guilty of such failure as no ordinary doctor of ordinary skill would be guilty of if acting with ordinary care.

Dr Hanley was found by the court not to have been negligent because the course he followed in treating his patient was one that an ordinary doctor might have followed if he had been acting with ordinary skill and ordinary care. This case was followed shortly afterwards by a similar case in England – the 'Bolam' case.

Case 15
The Bolam case[38]

In 1954, John Bolam was admitted to a psychiatric ward in Friern Hospital suffering from depression. It was decided that he should be treated with electroconvulsive therapy (ECT). When this treatment is given without muscle relaxant, the muscle spasms are associated with a slight risk of fracture.

When the treatment was administered, Dr Alfrey, in accordance with hospital policy did not use any muscle relaxant. Mr Bolam, who had not been warned of the risk of fracture, suffered bilateral fractures of the acetabula. He sued the hospital on the grounds that it was negligent in failing to administer a muscle relaxant, or warn him of the risks.

The expert witnesses for the two sides agreed that a large body of competent medical opinion was opposed to the use of muscle relaxants in ECT but disagreed about whether it was desirable or not to warn the patient of the risk of fracture.

In directing the jury the judge stated that 'The test is the standard of the ordinary skilled man exercising and professing to have that special skill; it is a well established law that it is sufficient if he exercises the ordinary skill of an ordinary competent man exercising that particular art'.

He went on 'A doctor is not guilty of negligence if he has acted in accordance with a practice accepted as proper by a responsible body of medical men skilled in that particular art...Putting it another way round, a doctor is not negligent if he is acting in accordance with such a practice, merely because there is a body of opinion that takes a contrary view.'

Again, the defendant was found not to have been negligent. The standard set by the court

in this case, as in *Hunter* v. *Hanley*, was that which a responsible body of medical opinion would accept. Some might argue that this allows the medical profession to set its own standards. It might also be argued that by requiring doctors to comply with the standard of the 'ordinary doctor' that their clinical freedom has been restricted.

At present, when reaching a view on what the 'ordinary doctor' would have done if acting with 'ordinary skill' and 'ordinary care', a court has to ask an 'ordinary competent man (or woman) exercising that particular art'. So what is the 'ordinary doctor' of 'ordinary skill' acting with 'ordinary care'? We know that this person cannot be a GP examining a patient's lumbar spine with the skill of a neurosurgeon – that would be 'extraordinary skill'. Equally, this person is not the radiologist examining mammograms after a liquid lunch with one eye on the television and who misses a lesion. Such an example could hardly be used to demonstrate a doctor exercising 'ordinary care'. With the number of people currently on the register held by the General Medical Council running into tens of thousands, how can a court judge what is 'ordinary'? Fortunately, Lord President Clyde went further and provided a tripartite test, which now forms the basis of every medical negligence case:[39]

- That there was a standard procedure or technique used in the circumstances faced by the allegedly negligent doctor
- That the allegedly negligent doctor departed from that standard procedure or technique
- That the departure was such that no doctor exercising ordinary care or skill would have adopted.

The expert witness

It is important that a practitioner from the same area of medicine is asked to provide evidence as to what 'usual and normal' practice is. Clearly it is unreasonable to expect a consultant psychiatrist to treat a patient who collapses with a cardiac arrest in the same way as a consultant in intensive care medicine would, and the law recognizes this. Disputes can arise between experts about what usual and normal practice is, and it is for the judge to decide which side has argued their position in the most logical fashion. As Lord Scarman[40] remarked:

> Differences of opinion and practice exist, and will always exist, in the medical as in other professions… I have to say that a judge's 'preference' for one body of distinguished professional opinion to another also professionally distinguished is not sufficient to establish negligence in a practitioner whose actions have received the seal of approval of those whose opinions, truthfully expressed, honestly held, were not preferred… Failure to exercise the ordinary skill of a doctor…is necessary.

However, the law has evolved considerably following *Bolitho* v. *Hackney Area Health Authority*,[41] in which it was held that for a judge to rely upon the opinion of a medical expert, the judge has to be satisfied that the expert's opinion has a logical basis. Although this might sound fairly nebulous, and perhaps obvious, it represents a turning point. Judges can now take an interventionalist approach in weighing up medical evidence and, if unsatisfied by the explanations of experts, reach their own conclusions. The days of unquestioning judicial deference to medical experts are numbered.

Some people have suggested that it would be better if the court itself appointed its own medical expert to advise the judge on these questions. It has also been suggested that the introduction of guidelines might assist courts in deciding what 'ordinary practice' is.

What do you think the advantages and disadvantages of the suggestions would be?

Harm

Before any claim can be successful it is necessary to establish that the negligence caused the loss or suffering for which compensation is claimed. In short, a causal link must be shown. In some cases – even where the breach of duty is obvious or is admitted – it can be very difficult to link these two elements. This point is illustrated in the Scottish case of *Kay's Tutor* v. *Ayrshire and Arran Health Board*.[42]

Case 16
Penicillin overdose

A young child was admitted to hospital with meningitis. He was treated with penicillin. Unfortunately, he was given a very large overdose that resulted in him having convulsions. After he recovered his health, he was found to be profoundly deaf. His father sued on his behalf for compensation for his loss of hearing. It was clear that administration of such a large overdose was in breach of the duty of care owed to him by the hospital. However, the court heard from various experts that the cause of the boy's deafness was due to the meningitis and the court held that 'The medical evidence simply failed to prove any causal link between the penicillin overdose and the deafness'.

As a consequence, no damages were awarded for the loss of hearing, even although the administering of the overdose was clearly negligent. Therefore, in establishing causation, persons bringing a claim must establish 'on the balance of probability' that the doctor's alleged negligence contributed materially to their injury or loss.

Compensation

The only form of remedy a civil court can provide is money, known as 'damages'. These damages are supposed to compensate the patient for loss (e.g. pain and/or loss of income and job prospects); they are not supposed to punish the doctor or the doctor's employer. Suppose that the architect we considered earlier designs a garage for you and it falls down shortly after completion, crushing your car. If it can be shown that the architect was negligent in carrying out the work, then it seems reasonable that he or she should compensate you for the cost of rebuilding the garage and repairing or replacing your car. However, it is much more difficult to think about how someone can be compensated for the loss of a leg, the loss of their sight or the loss of a child. If the faculty that is lost means more to one person than another, should they be compensated differently? Is the leg of a professional footballer worth more than that of an office worker, or the eyesight of an artist worth more than that of a down-and-out alcoholic?

Spend some time discussing with colleagues how you could quantify such losses if they were due to medical negligence.

Inquiries into sudden deaths and fatal accidents

There has been a long tradition of state officials taking an interest in sudden and suspicious deaths.[43] Interestingly, these long-established forums of accountability could offer ways of thinking about systems failures and the lessons to be learned from them, rather than simply seeking to apportion blame to individuals.

When a person's death is sudden or unexpected, or occurs in certain special circumstances (Table 4.2), procedures exist to examine the circumstances surrounding the events related to the death. On occasions this will include the deaths of patients who were under the care of a doctor or hospital prior to death. In countries with a common law tradition, such as England, Wales and Northern

---

Table 4.2

Deaths that should be reported to the coroner or procurator fiscal

- Uncertified deaths
- Suspicious or violent deaths, including accidents
- Deaths as a result of suicide
- Deaths as a result of drowning, fire or explosions
- Deaths caused by neglect, hypothermia or drug abuse
- Infant deaths, including sudden infant death syndrome
- Deaths of foster children
- Deaths that occur within 24 hours of emergency admission to hospital or within 24 hours of a surgical operation
- Deaths where medical negligence is alleged
- Deaths in police custody or prison
- Deaths caused by shipping, rail or aircraft accidents
- Deaths caused by industrial disease or poisoning
- Deaths caused by accidents at work

Ireland, such deaths are reported to the coroner, who will undertake enquiries before conducting an inquest. In Scotland a separate system exists.

Fatal accident inquiries

In Scotland, when a death is thought to be reportable, doctors should contact the procurator fiscal. If the death has resulted from an accident at work, or where the death has occurred when a person is in legal custody, an inquiry is usually mandatory. In other circumstances, a fatal accident inquiry (FAI) can be held on a discretionary basis. Such an inquiry will be held 'if it appears to the Lord Advocate to be expedient in the public interest…that an inquiry…should be held into the circumstances of the death on the grounds that it was sudden, suspicious or unexplained, or has occurred in circumstances such as to give rise to serious public concern'.[44] One of the purposes of FAIs is to identify ways of working that, if they were allowed to continue or recur, would be prejudicial to the health and safety of the public.

FAIs, which are held in public, are presided over by a sheriff and all interested parties can attend. It is the job of the procurator fiscal to set out the facts of the case before the sheriff by questioning relevant witnesses on oath. Doctors and other healthcare workers might be required to appear and answer questions about their involvement in the care of patients. If necessary, they can be represented by a lawyer. Arranging representation at FAIs is one of the main tasks of the medical defence organizations (MDOs), and members are advised to contact their MDO if they become aware that they are likely to have to attend an FAI.

Once all the evidence has been heard, the sheriff produces a written 'determination' in which he or she states where and when the death or accident took place and the cause or causes of death and of any accident resulting in death. The sheriff can also comment on reasonable precautions whereby the death might have been avoided, any defects in a system of working that contributed to the death or accident and 'any other facts which are relevant to the circumstances of the death' (Table 4.3).

This means that doctors who have been involved in designing systems for the delivery of care, perhaps by drawing up protocols or delegating duties to others, could be made to account for the way they made their decisions in such a forum. It also allows the

sheriff to identify systems that are faulty and that can be improved. Yet various decisions following inquiries have demonstrated that a sheriff's determination is not to be used to apportion blame or 'try' those connected with the death.

Coroners' inquiries

In England and Wales, the coroner enquires into notifiable deaths, most of which are reported by the police, the Registrar of Births and Deaths or doctors. A similar system exists in Northern Ireland to allow coroner's inquests to be held. Once the coroner's preliminary investigation (which usually involves receiving statements from those involved) is complete, he or she can decide to hold an inquest that can, in some circumstances, involve a jury. A coroner must sit with a jury for deaths that occur in police custody or are related to industrial, shipping, rail or aircraft accidents. Unlike the Scottish system, where the roles of the sheriff and procurator fiscal are separate, the coroner is the one who investigates the circumstances of the death, presents the evidence at the inquest and examines the witnesses, and either returns a verdict or assists the jury in doing so. The relatives can be represented by a lawyer, as can doctors if necessary. It is sound practice for doctors to inform their medical defence organization if they are summoned to give evidence to a coroner's inquest, especially if medical negligence is being suggested.

The inquests are held in public, although the public can be excluded from all or part of the inquest if the coroner considers that this is in the national interest. At the end of the inquest a verdict is reached that includes:

- the name of the deceased (if known)
- details of the injury or disease causing death
- the time, place and circumstances at or in which injury was sustained
- the conclusions of the jury/coroner as to the death

Table 4.3
Fatal Accidents and Sudden Deaths (Scotland) Act 1976 – the Sheriff's determination[44]

- Where and when the death and any accident resulting in the death took place
- Cause or causes of death or the accident resulting in the death
- The cause or causes of any accident resulting in the death
- The reasonable precautions, if any, whereby the death and any accident resulting in the death might have been avoided
- The defect, if any, in any system of working which contributed to the death or any accident resulting in the death
- Any other facts which are relevant to the circumstances of the death

- particulars required by the Registration Acts (e.g. address, sex, maiden name, occupation of the deceased, etc.)

The coroner is not allowed to frame a verdict in such a way as to name a person responsible for criminal liability; however, a verdict of 'unlawful killing' can be returned and the case referred to the Crown Prosecution Service.[45] Other possible verdicts include:

- natural causes
- accidental death or misadventure
- suicide
- neglect
- open verdict – where there is insufficient evidence to determine the cause of death. In this situation the inquest can be resumed later if more evidence comes to light.

Both approaches for examining sudden and unexpected deaths provide frameworks for looking at possible errors and lessons to be learnt from them that may lead to genuine improvements in health care provision.

> Try to find the time to attend an FAI or coroner's inquest. Think about what questions you would ask and how you would ask them.

The criminal justice system

Doctors, like all other members of society, are subject to the rule of law and can be subject to criminal prosecution if the prosecuting authorities believe an offence has been committed. The most notorious case in living memory is that of the GP Harold Shipman, who was found guilty of murdering a number of his patients and sentenced to life imprisonment.[46] Prosecutions for criminal offences are thankfully rare against doctors but prosecuting authorities will consider

charging doctors with manslaughter (or culpable homicide in Scotland) if they 'showed such disregard for the life and safety of others as to amount to a crime against the State and conduct deserving of punishment'.[47]

Case 17
Anaesthetic disaster

In 1987 a 33-year-old man underwent an operation to repair a detached retina. During the procedure, the tube from the ventilator to the patient's mouth became disconnected; the anaesthetist did not notice this. The patient's blood pressure and pulse fell. The anaesthetist's response to the fall in the patient's blood pressure and pulse rate was to assume the monitor was faulty. The patient then suffered a cardiac arrest, at which point the surgeon noticed that the tube was disconnected. The patient died later of irreversible brain damage. Expert evidence at the trial indicated that any competent anaesthetist looking after the patient would have realized total disconnection within seconds.

The anaethetist was sentenced to 6 months' imprisonment suspended for 12 months.[48]

Another recent manslaughter case concerned two junior doctors.

Case 18
Cytotoxic error

In 1993 a junior house officer (JHO) and a senior house officer (SHO) were convicted of manslaughter at Birmingham Crown Court following an error in administering cytotoxic drugs to a 16-year-old patient with leukaemia.[49]

The patient was attending for cytotoxic therapy in the form of monthly intravenous injections of vincristine and bi-monthly intrathecal injections of methotrexate. An error arose when the patient attended for both injections in February 1990. A red box was delivered to the ward by the hospital pharmacy and placed on a trolley set up for the lumbar puncture. This box contained two syringes, one filled with methotrexate and the other with vincristine. Both the box and the individual syringes were clearly labelled with details of the drug and route of administration.

The JHO was reluctant to do the procedure because of his inexperience and the SHO was sent to supervise him. Confusion arose because the JHO thought the SHO would supervise the whole procedure, whereas the SHO thought he was supervising only the lumbar puncture. Because of this misunderstanding between the doctors, when the needle was in the patient's spine the SHO handed the JHO the wrong syringe and vincristine was wrongly injected into the patient's spine, with fatal results.

Their convictions for manslaughter (they both received 9 months, suspended for 12 months) were quashed on appeal. Sadly, despite the high profile of this case, this fatal error has recurred in UK hospitals.

Analyse this serious error from both the 'person' and 'system' perspective.

The General Medical Council

An Act of Parliament established the General Medical Council (GMC) in 1858. Its purpose was to set up and maintain a register of medical practitioners.

In effect, to be a 'doctor' means that one is a medical practitioner on the register held by the GMC. The reverse is also true: if one ceases to be on the register one also ceases to be a 'doctor'. Removal or suspension from the register is the main sanction that the GMC has, which it will consider using in certain circumstances.

The GMC, which is comprised of a majority of doctors and a minority of lay people, is a self-regulatory body. It describes its role as 'protecting patients and guiding doctors'. To fulfil this function, the GMC is involved in setting standards of behaviour for doctors

and issuing guidance to doctors in a number of areas, including 'good medical practice', 'maintaining good medical practice', 'consent to treatment', 'confidentiality' and other 'duties of a doctor'.[50] It is wise for all doctors to be familiar with the contents of this advice. The GMC also monitors the quality of undergraduate training and regularly visits medical schools. In the future, the GMC is likely to take a greater role in ensuring the standard of practising doctors.

The GMC also investigates complaints and concerns about the conduct, performance or health of doctors. Before looking at how it holds doctors accountable in these areas, it is worthwhile considering what the GMC states are the core duties of a doctor:

- Make the care of the patient the first concern
- Treat every patient politely and considerately
- Respect patients' dignity and privacy
- Listen to patients and respect their views
- Give patients information in a way they can understand
- Respect the rights of patients to be fully involved in discussions about their case
- Keep professional knowledge and skills up to date
- Recognize the limits of individual professional competence
- Be honest and trustworthy
- Respect and protect confidential information
- Ensure personal beliefs do not prejudice patients' care
- Act quickly to protect patients at risk from a colleague who is not fit to practise
- Avoid abusing his/her position as a doctor
- Work with colleagues in the way that best serves the patient interest
- Never discriminate unfairly against patients or colleagues
- Be prepared to justify actions to patients and colleagues.

This list of duties would appear at first sight to be perfectly laudable but, as with most lists of rights and duties, problems can arise when different items on the list come into conflict. For example, in Chapter 3 (p. 44–51) we considered how doctors should act when they believe that confidential information should be disclosed in a patient's best interest but the patient refuses. Should doctors 'respect and protect' the confidential information or should 'the care of the patient be the first concern'? Likewise, in a world of expanding information, how 'up to date' does a doctor's 'professional knowledge and skills' have to be?

It is to be noted that the GMC still talks about 'patients', and also that it emphasizes that doctors have a duty to be prepared to justify their actions to patients and colleagues.

- Compare the 'duties of a doctor' listed above with the core values of your medical school.
- Consider the problems associated with core value and duty statements.

The GMC has powers to require doctors to be accountable to it in three main areas:

- health
- performance
- professional conduct.

Complaints can be made to the GMC by patients or their relatives, professional colleagues, employing authorities and Trusts and community health councils. In addition, the police automatically notify the GMC if a doctor is convicted of a criminal offence.

When a complaint is received by the GMC it is screened by a medical member and/or a lay member, who consider the seriousness of the matter and whether the case should be rejected, referred to the health screener, referred to the preliminary proceedings committee on the grounds of conduct or referred for assessment under performance.

Health procedures

Where a doctor's health is causing a risk to patients, the aim of these procedures is to allow the doctor to be treated and return to unrestricted practice, while at the same time also protecting patients. To achieve this, the doctor is invited to undergo an assessment, which could include a medical examination, by a doctor appointed by the GMC. The report will indicate the steps needed to restore the doctor to full health and any restrictions on his or her practice that are required to safeguard patients in the meantime. There is usually a period of monitoring by a medical supervisor until the doctor returns to unrestricted practice. These procedures are conducted in strict confidence. Occasionally a doctor's health is such that a return to practice is not possible, or a doctor might fail to comply with the suggested procedures. In these circumstances, the case can be referred to the GMC's Health Committee, which has the power to impose restrictions on the doctor's registration or to suspend him or her from the medical register.

Performance procedures

Where the screener considers that issues relating to a doctor's competence have been raised, the doctor might be asked to undergo a process of assessment. Such assessments are carried out by an assessment panel and usually involve a visit to the doctor's place of practice, where the assessors interview the doctor and his or her colleagues. The assessors might also observe the doctor at work and examine the medical records of his or her patients. In addition, the doctor could also be required to attend an assessment centre for an objective structured clinical examination (OSCE). Following the assessment, a report will be prepared identifying any weaknesses in the doctor's performance and suggesting remedial actions that should be undertaken, such as areas of retraining or further study. There will then follow a reassessment.

Where remedial action fails to significantly improve performance, or where a doctor's level of performance is so poor that it is felt patients are seriously at risk, or where a doctor refuses to cooperate with an assessment, the case will be referred to the Committee on Professional Performance. This committee, at which the doctor can be legally represented, can impose conditions on the doctor's registration or suspend his or her name from the register.

Conduct procedures

If the screener considers that a complaint raises issues of 'serious professional misconduct' the case will be referred to the Preliminary Proceedings Committee. This committee reviews the complaint, any evidence that has been collected and any comments the doctor in question has made. It will then decide whether to:

- take no further action
- send the doctor a written warning
- refer the case to the Committee, or to the Committee on Professional Health or Performance
- refer the case to the Professional Conduct Committee – if the case is serious enough the doctor can be suspended on an interim basis until a full hearing takes place.

The Professional Conduct Committee, which decides whether the doctor is guilty of serious professional misconduct, follows procedures similar to a court of law. Hearings are conducted in public, the process is adversarial and lawyers represent both sides. Evidence is given on oath and both sides can call and cross-examine witnesses. If the case against a doctor is found by the committee to have been proven it can:

- admonish the doctor
- impose conditions on the doctor's registration
- suspend the doctor's registration
- remove the doctor's name from the medical register.

Appeals

A doctor has the right of appeal to the Judicial Committee of the Privy Council.

The future of self-regulation

At present, the GMC will hear about doctors it has permitted onto its register only if there is a reason to question whether they are still fit to practise. In response to the changes in public and political demand, it is likely that this approach will be turned around entirely and, in the future, doctors on the medical register will have to justify their continued presence on the register. Steps are already being taken to devise a system that will require practitioners to amass evidence of their clinical competence in order that they can be 'reaccredited' on a regular basis. It is likely that doctors in all areas of medicine will be expected to compile a portfolio of information about their performance and continuing professional development, which will be subject to periodic peer review as part of a system of quality assurance.

- What measures do you think it would be appropriate to include in such a portfolio?
- Should complaints and claims against individuals be included?

It is to be hoped that such a system will identify doctors with problems at an early stage, thereby reducing the risk to patients and improving the chances of helping the practitioners to overcome their difficulties. Where problems cannot be resolved locally, the powers of the GMC, described above, can be deployed. As the clinical governance movement develops more sophisticated tools for assessing quality, it is likely that the outcome of audit will feed into the process of reaccreditation.

One of the recommendations included in the report of the Bristol Royal Infirmary Inquiry was that there should be an overarching body for the regulation of the healthcare professions. It seems likely that the government will establish a Council for the Regulation of Healthcare Professions in the foreseeable future. Such a development would streamline the way in which doctors, nurses, pharmacists and various other groups of professionals are educated, revalidated and disciplined.

> Can you identify any sources of potential conflict between individual accountability and the responsibility of systems?

Other registering bodies

A number of organizations exist to regulate the other healthcare professions. These bodies also maintain registers of members and have similar procedures to investigate allegations of serious professional misconduct or infamous conduct of those on their registers. Again, the main sanction they have is removal or suspension of an individual's registration. Some, but not all, will also take an interest in the health problems of those registered with them. Table 4.4 summarizes these organizations.

The role of medical defence organizations

As the concept of professional accountability emerged at the end of the nineteenth century,

Table 4.4
The different regulatory healthcare bodies

Profession	Regulatory body	Conduct	Health	Performance
Doctors	General Medical Council	+	+	+
Dentists	General Dental Council	+	+	−
Nurses, midwives and health visitors	United Kingdom Central Council for Nursing, Midwifery and Health Visiting	+	+	+
Pharmacists	Royal Pharmaceutical Society of Great Britain	+	−	−
Physiotherapists	Chartered Society of Physiotherapists	+	+	−
Homoeopaths	Society of Homoeopaths	+	−	+
Osteopaths	General Osteopathic Council	+	−	+
Chiropractors	British Chiropractic Association	+	−	−
Opticians	The General Optical Council	+	−	−
Speech therapists	Royal College of Speech and Language Therapists	+	−	+
Acupuncturists	British Acupuncture Council	+	+	−
Chiropodists, dietitian, occupational therapists, orthoptics, radiographers and art therapists	Council of Professions Supplementary to Medicine	+	−	−

+, the regulatory body regulates this aspect of professional behaviour; − the regulatory body does not regulate this aspect of professional behaviour.

three mutual organizations were founded to offer both professional indemnity and support and advice to doctors and dentists. The Medical Defence Union was founded in 1888 and was followed by the Medical Protection Society in 1892 and the Medical and Dental Defence Union of Scotland in 1902. One of the strengths of the way these organizations are structured is their ability to exercise discretion over the way they help members. In the rapidly changing environment of accountability they are able to modify their services to fit the needs of their members. Since 1990, doctors working in NHS hospitals are covered by the provisions of 'crown indemnity', which means that any damages awarded in a civil claim against them are paid for from NHS funds.[52] Representation before the GMC, inquiries and disciplinary hearings, however, are becoming an increasingly important part of the MDOs' work with doctors in all areas of medicine.

By drawing on the experience obtained from reviewing medical errors and misadventures, the MDOs are increasingly developing clinical risk management services for their members. Before briefly looking at the subject of risk management, we will consider the right of patients to access information about themselves and their health.

Medical records – the patient's right to know

The knowledge and skills doctors and healthcare workers possess allow them to acquire information about other people's health of which those individuals would not otherwise necessarily be aware. For example, interpretation of the presenting signs and symptoms, or analysis of test results, can allow a doctor to learn that a patient has a condition that has implications for that individual's future. The question that arises is to whom does this information belong and who should have rights over it. The issue of the confidentiality of this information is discussed in Chapter 3 (p. 44–51).

In the past, information relating to a patient's health was generally seen as being in the safekeeping of doctors, who would disclose only that information they considered the patient 'required' to know and was in the 'best interests' of the patient. The past few years have witnessed a significant shift in attitudes towards the ownership and control of this information. The Data Protection Act of 1984 was a landmark step in promoting the rights of individuals to have access to information held about them. Although this first piece of legislation applied to information held on computer systems, which were rapidly expanding at that time, there shortly afterwards followed the Access to Health Records Act (1990), which introduced for the first time the right of patients to request access to their health records. Prior to this, patients had no right to demand to see what was written about them in their records.

From March 2000, individuals have had rights of access to their health records, whether computerized or manual, and whenever they were made under the Data Protection Act 1998. In just over 10 years there has been a considerable swing in the law in favour of individuals having rights over information concerning them. Indeed, there are now moves to introduce 'smart cards' to allow patients to carry around their own medical records. The cards, which are being discussed by the government's panel on 'patient empowerment', are designed to allow patients to find information about themselves and to make doctors more accountable.[52] This represents another aspect to the changing environment in which doctors and patients relate to one another.

Risk management and clinical governance

To lose one parent may be regarded as a misfortune; to lose both looks like carelessness.

Oscar Wilde[53]

At the risk of sounding flippant, this quote highlights a truth in medicine that whilst misfortunes and accidents do occur, it is important that steps are taken to learn from such incidents to ensure similar problems do not recur, if they are avoidable. The discipline of risk management that has been developed in the insurance and financial industries is increasingly being applied to medicine. By setting in place a system that encourages an open review of critical incidents, near misses and complaints, together with a process of audit of outcome and performance, healthcare providers can identify working practices that needlessly expose patients, staff or others to risks. As we have observed, to err is human and, as society comes to realize that this applies to doctors, the demand that doctors never make mistakes becomes unsustainable. It is important that a 'no blame' culture is fostered so that doctors and nurses feel encouraged to report such incidents. By monitoring the results of clinical audit and other strategic information, the process of risk management allows those responsible for the delivery of the service to develop an effective system of clinical governance.

Different people define clinical governance in subtly different ways, but it is helpful to think of it as a system that asks the following questions 'Are we doing the right thing?', 'Are we doing it right?', 'How are we checking that we are doing it right?' and 'What are we doing about it?'.[54] When considering how this can be achieved in healthcare it is again helpful to look beyond medicine to learn from the experience of other 'high reliability organizations'. As Reason[55] observes:

> Although some unsafe acts in any sphere are egregious, the vast majority are not. In aviation maintenance – a hands-on activity similar to medical practice in many respects – some 90% of quality lapses were judged as blameless. Effective risk management depends crucially on establishing a reporting culture. Without a detailed analysis of mishaps, incidents, near misses, and 'free lessons', we have no way of uncovering recurrent error traps or of knowing where the 'edge' is until we fall over it. The complete absence of such a reporting culture within the Soviet Union contributed crucially to the Chernobyl disaster. Trust is a key element of a reporting culture and this, in turn, requires the existence of a just culture – one possessing a collective understanding of where the line should be drawn between blameless and blameworthy actions. Engineering a just culture is an essential early step in creating a safe culture.

Another serious weakness of the person approach [discussed above] is that by focusing on the individual origins of error it isolates unsafe acts from their system context. As a result, two important features of human error tend to be overlooked. Secondly, far from being random, mishaps tend to fall into recurrent patterns. The same set of circumstances can provoke similar errors, regardless of the people involved. The pursuit of greater safety is seriously impeded by an approach that does not seek out and remove the error provoking properties within the system at large.

A number of initiatives in medicine[56] seek to develop this approach by analysing 'adverse incidents' and 'near misses' in a confidential and supportive environment to maximize the potential benefit in terms of improving systems and behaviour.

Record keeping

When a doctor has to review the care of a patient, a clear set of contemporaneous notes, which details the author's investigations, observations and conclusions, is invaluable. We have discussed a wide range of forums in which doctors and other healthcare workers increasingly have to be prepared to offer accounts of their decisions and, in these situations, good records might be the only evidence they can call on for support. We will now consider some practical suggestions that will assist in the process of ensuring that good quality records will be available when required.

There is often a considerable time lapse between an incident and the professionals involved having to give an account of their involvement in it. Therefore, even for those with excellent memories, it can be almost impossible to recall precisely the sequence of events and the thought processes that were taking place at the time. For this reason the most helpful aid professionals can have to turn to when they are held to account is a good quality, contemporaneous record of events. In making these observations we hope that readers will not lose sight of the fact that the purpose of keeping records is primarily to aid patient care, by allowing members of the healthcare team to share information about their patients. However, the features of good record keeping described below apply equally to their clinical and forensic use. As one cannot predict which cases will be discussed, perhaps years later, it is good practice to get into the habit of keeping records that are:

- Contemporaneous: notes should be written as close in time to the events they describe as possible. Inevitably the recollection of events fades and becomes distorted by time. Court and other tribunals place considerable weight on contemporaneous records
- Dated and timed: in trying to reconstruct the flow of events at a later date, this information can be very important in establishing what happened and who did what when
- Legible and signed: notes are of limited value if others cannot read them; even worse if the writer cannot either! It is also important that the author of the records can be identified

- Logical: notes that make clear what the doctor was presented with, the questions that were asked, what findings were made, what thoughts these factors gave rise to and what the management plan was, will not only add weight to the impression that the writer is a logical and competent practitioner but also assist the individual recall their involvement in the case at a later date. Where appropriate, a sketch can speak volumes
- Consistent: it is vital that clinicians are consistent in their use of abbreviations and form of note taking wherever possible. First, this will be of great assistance to colleagues and, second, the actions and assumptions of such a consistent practitioner are usually easier to defend.

When things go wrong, as they inevitably will for all practitioners, it is often a good exercise to write down as full a report of the incident as possible. Where the contemporaneous record is deficient, this is the appropriate place to record missing information and comments. It is vital that the clinical records are not added to or modified in a way that could be construed as tampering with evidence. To do so risks attracting accusations of dishonesty, which invariably make a bad situation very much worse!

Conclusions: The future – a change in culture

If healthcare professionals are to learn from their mistakes and to use the lessons to be found in examining errors to improve the service they provide, then a significant change in culture is required. It has been suggested that a move away from the current 'blame culture' in which individuals are subject to criticism and punishment is necessary before doctors and other healthcare workers will feel able openly to discuss their errors and near misses. There appear to be lessons to be learnt from other professions, such as airline pilots, who have a system that allows them freely to report errors in a confidential and safe way that puts the rights of future passengers above those of past ones by denying those affected by errors the opportunity of recovering compensation.

The current challenge facing society is to develop a culture within which the quality of healthcare is assured and healthcare professionals are able to concentrate on improving this quality through life-long learning and by being able to evaluate and develop their performance. Appropriate systems of accountability will be part of this system.

To conclude:

- All doctors must be prepared to explain their actions
- Good communication between doctors and patients reduces the risk of complaints
- Trust between doctors and patients, both at the level of the individual and the level of society, is important and can be supported by clear systems of accountability
- Most healthcare professions are self-regulating, although this is currently being challenged
- Most methods of accountability focus on the individual rather than the system
- Everyone makes mistakes and it is often the best people who make the worst mistakes – error is not the monopoly of an unfortunate few
- Tensions exist between the demands of consumerism and the autonomy of doctors; the concept of partnership is becoming popular
- If improvements in the safety of patients are to be achieved, a change in culture is required
- Individuals' rights of access to information are increasing and will lead to a greater need to explain and inform patients and their carers about what is proposed before obtaining consent

- The regulatory framework for health professionals is complex and set to change
- The only thing certain about the future is its uncertainty.

Notes and references

1 The Times. Friday 2 June 2000.
2 Jean Ritchie QC chaired an independent inquiry into the conduct of a consultant gynaecologist. The report stated that NHS consultants were treated 'like gods' in a 'closed atmosphere where there was, and probably still is, a culture of junior doctors being reluctant to criticise their seniors'. The report called for wide-ranging changes to the way the General Medical Council disciplines doctors.
3 Department of Health. A first class service: quality in the new NHS (HSC (98)113). London: Department of Health; 1998.
4 Smith R. All changed, changed utterly. Br Med J 1998; 316:1917–1918.
5 Further details are available: www.Bristol-Inquiry.org.uk
6 *Thake* v. *Maurice* [1986] 1 All ER 497.
7 Downie RS, Macnaughton J. Clinical judgement. Oxford: Oxford University Press; 2000.
8 Beresford NW, Evans TW. Legal safeguards for the audit process. Br Med J 1999; 319:654–656.
9 Fox TF. Professional freedom. Lancet 1951; ii:115–119.
10 Drummond H. Power: creating it, using it. London: Kogan Page; 1991.
11 Butler JR, Vaile MSB. Health and health services. London: Routledge & Kegan Paul; 1984.
12 Issac-Henry K, Painter C. The management challenges in local government – emerging trends. Local Government Studies 1991; 17(3):69–89.
13 Issac-Henry K et al. Management in the public sector – challenge and change. London: International Thomson Business Press; 1997.
14 Stewart J, Clark M. The public service organisation: issues and dilemmas. Public Administration 1987; 65(2):161–177.
15 Downie RS, Macnaughton J. Clinical judgement. Oxford: Oxford University Press; 2000.
16 Charles C et al. Shared decision making in the medical encounter: what does it mean? (or it takes two to tango). Social Science and Medicine 1997; 49:651–661.
17 Emanuel EJ, Emanuel LL. Four models of the physician-patient relationship. JAMA 1992; 267:2221–2226.
18 Charles C. et al. What do we mean by partnership in making decisions about treatment? Br Med J 1999; 319:780–782.

19 Graves D. Shake-up call on bungling doctor. Daily Telegraph, Friday 2 June 2000.

20 Guardian, Friday 14 July 2000.

21 Potter J. Consumerism and the public sector: how well does the coat fit. Public Administration 1987; 66(2):149–164.

22 Coulter A. Paternalism or partnership? Br Med J 1999; 319:719–720.

23 Tayside Health Council Annual Report 1999. Available from Scottish Health on the Web website: www.show.scot.nhs.uk/thc

24 Secretary of State for Health. Saving lives: our healthier nation. London: HMSO (Cm 4386); 1999.

25 Hobbes T. Leviathan. Originally published 1651; reprinted CB Macpherson (Ed.). Leviathan. Middlesex: Penguin; 1968.

26 Locke J. The second treatise of civil government. An essay concerning the true origin, extent, and end of civil government. Originally published in 1690 and reprinted in: Laslett P. Two treatises of government (1690). Cambridge: Cambridge University Press; 1967.

27 Jain A, Ogden J. General practitioners' experiences of patients' complaints: qualitative study. Br Med J 1999; 318:1596–1599.

28 Reason J. Human error: models and management. Br Med J 2000; 320:768–770.

29 Reason J. Human error: models and management. Br Med J 2000; 320:768–770.

30 Department of Health. Being heard: the report of a review committee on NHS complaints procedures (D016/BH/10M, HSSH J032708). London: DoH; 1984.

31 Jain A, Ogden J. General practitioners' experiences of patients' complaints: qualitative study. Br Med J 1999; 318:1596–1599.

32 Rodger J. Personal communication.

33 Health Service Ombudsman. A guide to the work of the Health Service Ombudsman. London: Office of the Health Service Commissioner; 1996.

34 Dickson RH. Medical and dental negligence. Edinburgh: T&T Clark; 1997.

35 'Solatium' is defined as compensation for pain and suffering arising from the personal injuries, from the time of the injury up to the date of bringing the action and for the future.

36 *Hatcher* v. *Black* [1954] CLY 2289.

37 *Hunter* v. *Hanley* [1955] SC 200, 1955 SLT 213.

38 *Bolam* [1957] 2 All ER 118, [1957] 1WLR 582.

39 *Maynard* [1955] SC 200, 1955 SLT 213.

40 *Maynard* v. *West Midlands Regional Health Authority* [1985] 1 All ER 635.

41 *Bolitho* v. *Hackney Health Authority* 1997.

42 *Kay's Tutor* v. *Ayrshire and Arran Health Board* [1987] 2 All ER 417.

43 Carmichael IHB. Sudden deaths and fatal accident inquiries. Edinburgh: W Green and Son; 1986.

44 Fatal Accidents and Sudden Deaths Inquiry (Scotland) Act 1976.

45 Coroners Rules 1984 (SI 1984 No. 552).

46 Britain's worst serial killer. The Times. Tuesday 1 Febuary 2000.

47 *R.* v. *Bateman* [1925] 94 LJKB 791.

48 *R.* v. *Adomako* [1994] 5 Med LR 277.

49 *R.* v. *Prentice and Sullman* [1993] 4 Med LR 304.

50 Copies of the GMC's publications are available from the GMC website: www.gmc.org.uk

51 NHS Circular 1989 (PCS/32). Reprinted in Jones MA, Morris AE Blackstone's Statutes on Medical Law, 2nd edn. London: Blackstone Press Ltd, 1999.

52 Daily Telegraph. Monday 17 April 2000.

53 Wilde O. The importance of being earnest. London: Penguin Books, 2000.

54 Bulstrode C. In: Hospital Doctor 15 April 1999.

55 Reason J. Human error: models and management. Br Med J 2000; 320:768–770.

56 Pringle M. The inter-relationship between continuing professional development, clinical governance and revalidation for individual general practitioners. J Clin Governance 1999; 7(3):102–105.

5

The end of life

Introduction

Some of the most significant challenges in medical ethics occur at the end of life. This is always a serious and often a distressing time. Everyone who comes into contact with the dying and the bereaved is unquestionably touched by the experience (Fig. 5.1). Whereas end of life issues might be more pressing for those healthcare providers who work regularly with dying people, at some point in their careers, all medical professionals must confront the challenge of postponing death, or making the dying process as humane as possible. Because of the significance of this time in life, the ethical problems associated with it can be especially sensitive and the outcomes all the more important.

Case 19
When love broke the law...[1]

In 1985, James Brady learned that he had inherited the gene for Huntington's disease, a degenerative illness of the central nervous system. The gene for Huntington's is dominant, which means that someone carrying it will always be affected by it, and the disease cannot be cured.

James knew what kind of death he could expect: he, his brother Paul and their sister Margaret had already watched the disease claim the life of their mother some 20 years earlier, and he remembered the mental and physical deterioration that preceded her death.

The progress of the disease was relentless. Two years after his initial diagnosis, James was forced to give up his job as an engineer and, as his co-ordination deteriorated further, walking became increasingly difficult and his speech became slurred – a situation rendered all the

---

more humiliating by the fact that his condition was frequently mistaken for drunkenness. In 1993, James was admitted to a nursing home after collapsing in the street. He was soon bedridden and effectively helpless. It was around this time, according to his sister Margaret, that James began asking her for help in ending his life.

By Christmas 1995, James' wasted muscles were no longer under his control and his emaciated body was contorted by frequent convulsions. He had developed a variety of complications, including kidney and chest infections and liver damage, and he was barely able to swallow. In addition, he faced the indignity of relying upon his family and carers to attend to his most intimate personal needs. After spending Christmas with his family at Margaret's home, Paul was bathing James when his brother asked once more for help in ending his life.

The following evening, Paul gave James, who had already consumed a quantity of alcohol, around five or six times his prescribed dosage of temazepam. When he returned to the bedroom some time later, Paul found James still alive but unconscious, at which point he placed a pillow over his brother's face and suffocated him. He immediately informed the rest of the family what he had done.

This case illustrates how many moral questions arise in relation to death and dying. The most talked about of these is euthanasia, but it is not the only relevant issue. This chapter covers the following subjects:

- Euthanasia:
  - voluntary and involuntary euthanasia
  - passive and active euthanasia
  - the doctrine of the double effect
  - intentions

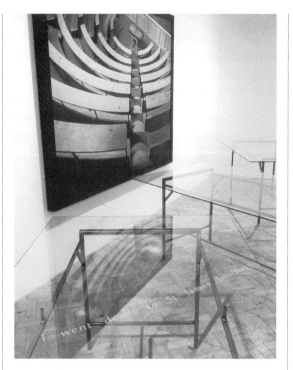

Figure 5.1
'Mysteries of the heart' Sue Brind and Jim Harold 1994. Commissioned by Book Works, London for 'The Reading Room' and shown at Camden Arts Centre, London. The title derives from an inscription in the Department of Human Anatomy at Oxford University, which, translated from Latin, reads: 'In this building the mysteries of the heart, the eyes, the limbs and the body can be studied one by one'. Etched into the glass table tops are these words from 'St James Infirmary' (© Joe Primrose 1930), which were sung by Louis Armstrong: 'I went down to St James Infirmary, To see my baby there, Stretched out on a long white table, So cold, so white, so bare'.

   – futile versus useful care
   – withholding and withdrawing treatment
   – advance directives or living wills
   – physician-assisted suicide
   – do not resuscitate orders
• Palliative care
• Sedation into unconsciousness.

The primary ethical concern facing Paul and James Brady was euthanasia.

Euthanasia

The term 'euthanasia' comes from the Greek meaning 'good death'. Taken in this sense, euthanasia is a fairly simple matter. However, it is complicated by considerations that go beyond just a good death. Euthanasia is sometimes known as mercy killing. In this sense, a number of issues complicate it, some of which will be discussed here. Broadly speaking, they include whether the patient requested or consented to the procedure, how it was performed and by whom.

Before reading any further, reflect on your own attitudes and understanding of euthanasia. Keep these in mind during the discussion that follows and return to them later to see if your ideas have been affected by the discussion.
    Even if you do not agree with them:

• List one or two reasons in support of euthanasia

• List one or two reasons against euthanasia

The case of James Brady is not unique. People regularly face fears associated with prolonged chronic illness, suffering, indignity and pain. A good number of people agree with James Brady's attitude – they prefer to die before their condition worsens beyond what they can endure. In James Brady's case, it is fairly clear that he sought to end his life and might have done so independently if he had been able. According to reports,[2] he valued his life enough to try to live as long as possible under his own terms. However, at some point this all became too much and he began to seek help in dying. He sought what he believed to be a good death with dignity and control.

Underlying the notion of the good death through mercy killing are ethical principles of autonomy, beneficence and non-maleficence. Supporters of euthanasia describe it as allowing a person to die whether by active or passive means for specific reasons. They seek to exercise their autonomy by ending suffering beyond endurance. This can take the form of uncontrollable pain or loss of dignity. The caregiver is then requested not to interfere with the patient's death or, as in the Brady case, actively to assist the patient to die. This is where the elements of beneficence and non-maleficence come to the fore. So long as the caregiver is performing the act of euthanasia with the intention of putting an end to the patient's suffering then, arguably, they will be helping the person or being beneficent. This is what Paul Brady claimed he was trying to do for his brother James. If the caregiver is removing the elements of care that are prolonging the patient's suffering then, the carer is being non-maleficent, or doing no harm, to the patient. It must be stated that the patient's autonomy can be preserved in this way if – and only if – the patient has requested or consented to the decision. It remains to be seen whether the claims of beneficence and non-maleficence are supportable.

Arguments for and against euthanasia will be covered below. Briefly, opponents of euthanasia claim that it cannot protect patient autonomy; after all, how can ending life preserve autonomy when it ultimately eliminates any possible future autonomy? Arguments against euthanasia state either that life is intrinsically valuable, as will be discussed below, or that it is never certain that a patient can voluntarily consent to euthanasia. Proponents disagree. They claim that euthanasia shows the ultimate respect for autonomy by helping someone to end a life that they find insufferable.

A number of distinctions have been established to help clarify the struggles. The most important ones are outlined below.

Voluntary versus involuntary euthanasia

Voluntary
The situation is voluntary when euthanasia is provided:

- at the request of a competent person
- with informed consent from a competent person
- by an advance directive (a 'living will') created when the person was competent.

In the case of James Brady there is little doubt that he had requested and desired euthanasia. He appeared to be competent when he made the request, as it was made only at the onset of the worst manifestations of the disease. His decision was informed because he knew from his mother's experience what he could expect. Nevertheless, questions still arise related to James Brady's competence at the time of his death, as we will see below. If a patient is not competent to realize the effects of their decision then the act cannot be voluntary.

Involuntary
The situation is involuntary when euthanasia is provided:

- for a patient who is unconscious
- for a patient who is incompetent to make an express wish in this regard
- otherwise without the patient's consent.

James Brady was conscious when his brother offered him the temazepam overdose; however, he was also drunk. Moreover, he was unconscious at the time of his death – suffocation administered by his brother Paul. Both these factors raise the possibility that this was a case of involuntary euthanasia. James was arguably incompetent at the time he accepted the overdose. He is likely to have been depressed by the effects the illness had on his life and by the prospects he faced. This could have been exaggerated by the alcohol, which is a known depressant. All of these features could have affected his judgement and caused him to accept the temazepam. Moreover, James was not conscious when his brother suffocated him with a pillow, and therefore could not have protested even if he wanted to. It is important to bear in mind that one can change one's mind about ending one's life, and people frequently do. Often, when patients claim they wish to die it can be a plea for help and a statement that they are not coping. In which case, less drastic measures should be sought to help them, bearing in mind that it is not always possible to do so and all patients have a right to refuse treatment. However, Paul Brady believed that he was acting in accordance with his brother's wishes on the evidence that James had made repeated requests before witnesses to be assisted to end his life.

Despite the possibilities described above, from what we know of the Brady case it is likely that this was truly an act of voluntary euthanasia. We know that James had persistently requested assistance in dying while he was competent and before witnesses. But there has long been debate regarding the possibility of consent to harm as an excuse for the accused. There are very good reasons for disallowing the victim's consent as an excuse for the perpetrator. Primarily because, more often than not, the victim of an actual crime will consent only out of coercion, therefore a crime has still been committed. For example, a murderer cannot be excused because a person submits to death rather than continued torture. Criminal courts do not recognize the excuse of consent under coercion or duress.

But criminal behaviour of this sort is not a perfect match to the euthanasia scenario. Here, the so called victim is asking for the hastening of death only because of uncontrollable pain and irredeemable loss of freedom and dignity due to incurable and life-threatening illness. There is no criminal coercion involved, no one is holding a gun to the patient's head to make him consent. Nevertheless, some will argue that there is a risk of a more subtle form of coercion. Patients could be led to agree to euthanasia rather than become a burden to their families or to society. This is one of the criticisms being levelled against the current situation in the Netherlands, where prosecuting authorities are unlikely to take action against doctors in euthanasia cases, provided certain safeguards are in place. At present, 'implicit coercion' is one of the strongest arguments against euthanasia. Arguments in favour of euthanasia say that, despite the possibility of coercion, it is necessary to pay heed to the reasoned requests of rational people. Otherwise we could argue against other sorts of appeals, such as the desire of a competent adult to smoke cigarettes. This raises questions of rational suicide and the right to die, which will be pursued in a later section of this chapter.

Passive versus active euthanasia

The type of act involved in euthanasia is also important. Theorists tend to distinguish between two types of acts of euthanasia: passive or active.

Passive

Passive euthanasia involves withholding treatment with the knowledge that applying it could save the person's life. The best example of this is refraining from performing resuscitation on patients with advanced stages of terminal cancer or patients in a persistent vegetative state (PVS). The reasoning behind this is that the patients are already dying from uncontrollable illness and resuscitation would only prolong the burden to them unnecessarily.

Active

Active euthanasia is the intentional administering of life-shortening medication to cause or accelerate death. Paul Brady performed exactly such an act when he gave his brother the temazepam and then placed a pillow over his head. Ideally, active euthanasia is performed only, if at all, at the request of voluntarily consenting patients.

It is notoriously difficult to distinguish between these two concepts. Passive euthanasia might be seen to include with-holding life-sustaining treatment such as nutrition and hydration. However, it is argued that this is more appropriately classified as active euthanasia because these two elements cannot be removed without knowingly causing the patient's death – no one can live very long without food and liquid. However, many physicians are more comfortable withholding nutrition and hydration when these only prolong suffering, than actively administering a lethal dose of medication. In this sense, withdrawal of nutrition and hydration is considered more passive than active by some people.

Doctrine of the double effect

> Permits an act which is foreseen to have both good and bad effects, provided: the act itself is good or at least indifferent; the good effect is not caused by the bad effect; a proportionate reason exists for causing the bad effect, e.g. morphine for pain may shorten life.[3]

Unintentional, although possibly foreseen, consequences of an act make it possible to praise rather than blame the actor, even though in other circumstances the same act or outcome would be considered blamewor-thy. Provided the intention is to be helpful, beneficent and non-maleficent, the conse-quences, it is said, can be overlooked. So the doctrine of the double effect is not a conse-quentialist position because it rests little judgement on the outcome of the act. The intentions are all that count and, in this sense, the doctrine is supportable by deontology.

The problem with the doctrine of the double effect is that it appears hypocritical. Opponents have severely criticized the

position because, as they point out, the actor who foresees the consequences of an action is acting intentionally and is therefore culpa-ble or responsible for the act and its outcome. It seems insincere to claim to be performing an act with the foreknowledge that both some bad effect 'x' and some good effect 'y' will occur, while at the same time stating that 'x' is not your intention, that you intend only 'y'.

Nevertheless, the position is widely accepted as a reasonable defence in certain circumstances. Also, many physicians embrace it as a better option to active euthanasia or physician-assisted suicide (see below). The doctrine of the double effect permits doctors to give dangerous or lethal doses of medication with the intention of relieving suffering, even though they know that doing so risks shortening the patient's life. They argue that this is more justifiable than active killing.

Intentions

The distinctions described above indicate the degree to which euthanasia is dependent upon intention. The intentions of the care-giver were considered in the Brady case to be the termination of James Brady's life. The judge's decision is described below.

Case 19 continued…
Paul Brady's intentions[4]

Paul was arrested and remanded in custody. He did not dispute that he had taken his brother's life, nor that he had done so deliberately.

Lord Macfadyen eventually elected to admonish Brady. In so doing, he made reference to 'a combination of powerful mitigating circumstances' that had influenced his decision, including the fact that Brady had acted out of 'compassion rather than from any malicious motive or any desire to make matters easier' for himself. He also referred to the fact that Paul's acts were carried out 'at his [James's] own earnest, and plainly heartfelt, request'.

Lord Macfadyen, however, was very careful to emphasize that the illegality of Paul Brady's actions had been recognized, and that it was only the 'exceptional' circumstances of this case that had deterred him from imposing a custodial sentence.

So Paul Brady was considered to have broken the law, and he was excused from punishment only because his intentions were believed to be morally justifiable. This was true only because Paul did not gain by his brother's death; only James stood to gain by ending his suffering and having his wishes respected. So far, except for a few countries, this is a common outcome of a euthanasia trial. Most often the actor is considered guilty of a crime but punishment varies from very weak, as it was for Paul Brady, to very strict, as in the case of Dr Jack Kevorkian in the US, who was eventually struck off and jailed for assisting in the deaths of multiple patients. Euthanasia is usually treated as a criminal act, and legislation in England and Scotland supports this decision. Hence, careful consideration of the consequences of assisting in an act of euthanasia must be made in advance. In certain cases criminal prosecution and punishment can be avoided if court authority is sought in advance. Consider the following case.

Case 20
Janet Johnstone

In 1996 the family and doctors of Janet Johnstone petitioned the court to remove the tube feeding that was keeping her alive. The petition was successful. Mrs Johnstone had been in a persistent vegetative state since January 1992, after taking an overdose of prescription drugs in an apparent suicide attempt. Tabloid newspaper reports suggested that a long history of abuse and depression were at the source of the attempt, which was not her first.[5]

Mrs Johnstone had been kept alive by tube feedings ever since, but doctors agreed that

---

there was no hope of recovery and that the intubation constituted unnecessary prolongation of her life. The media quoted her daughter Janet as saying that her mother had been dead for years.

After hearing the opinions of four neurologists regarding the hopelessness of the case, Lord Cameron of the Edinburgh Court of Session ruled 'that it was no longer in Janet Johnstone's best interest to keep her alive'.[6] The ruling permitted doctors to remove her feeding and hydration without fear of prosecution.

Futile versus useful care

These terms are used to distinguish between forms of treatment that are harmful and burdensome, as opposed to beneficial and tolerable. A treatment is liable to be considered futile or useless if it is unlikely to be successful. Doctors have no obligation to provide treatment they judge futile. It must, however, be noted that decisions about the futility of a treatment are frequently value based, and patients might have very different attitudes on the subject than professionals. For example, considerations ought to be made of the possible psychological benefits of treatments. This is a prime situation where discussion ought to precede the decision making.

Reference is occasionally made to extraordinary, heroic treatment, which is described as follows:

…extraordinary means should be understood as means that do not offer a reasonable chance of success and/or are foreseen to be excessively burdensome.[7]

In most cases, patients are well within their right of autonomy to reject all treatment they deem to be futile. If doctors disagree their only recourse is to persuade the patients to change their mind.

Withdrawing versus withholding treatment[8]

When treatment is believed to be burdensome to the patient it might be considered acceptable to withhold or withdraw it in order to alleviate suffering and prevent unnecessary prolongation of death:

> Good medical practice involves the alleviation of symptoms whilst causing the least harm. This in no way means that doctors should sustain life at all costs. Thus in issues of withholding or withdrawing medical treatment, the benefits to the patient have to be considered against possible harm, and the patient's wishes taken into account.[9]

Withholding

Refraining from administering treatment can be justified if the treatment is considered futile and unnecessarily burdensome. Otherwise, deliberate withholding of treatment is considered illegal and can lead to criminal prosecution and accusations of malpractice. Therefore it is best to withhold treatment only with consensus from the patient, patient's family and other healthcare professional.[10]

Withdrawing

Removal of treatment already begun for reasons of alleviating suffering and indignity related to burdensome and unnecessary treatment is more difficult than withholding treatment not begun. Hence, for example, there are fewer challenges to decisions not to insert feeding tubes than to seeking institutional or legal approval to withdraw a feeding tube after it has been inserted. Bearing this in mind, sometimes a test case is the only way to be certain that a procedure is truly futile.

Janet Johnstone's treatment was removed because it was perceived to be overly burdensome to prolong her life in PVS. However, it did take several court appeals and a great deal of time to permit the change of legislation that would allow her doctors to proceed. This decision was groundbreaking in Scotland, as was the similar judgement in England over the Tony Bland case in 1993. However, in neither country is the withdrawal of life-support measures sanctioned except with consultation and consensus from professional colleagues with appropriate expertise, and with court authorization.[11]

Advance directives or living wills

Although they still do not have any statutory authority in most countries, including the UK, advance directives (living wills) can be a useful means of ensuring one's values and wishes are considered even after one is unable to express them. Although they do not carry force of law, they can be, and have acted as, important clues to the potential or likely attitude an incapacitated patient might have towards the state of their health and diminished quality of life. Advance directives are a means of communicating anticipated attitudes and values. They are usually issued in writing, although verbal advance directives have been heeded in the past. Patients in a competent state prior to incapacitation can express their wishes regarding treatment, resuscitation and care. They can express their desire not to be kept alive via tube feeding if they are in an unalterable vegetative state, to be preserved from futile antibiotic treatment that could extend suffering or state that they do not wish to be resuscitated. In essence, an advance directive protects patients' rights to refuse treatment once they are no longer able to give informed consent.

More recently, living wills have been used to direct practitioners to perform procedures despite disabilities and perceived lack of quality of life. People with lasting disabilities, such as spina bifida and cerebral palsy, who are perfectly satisfied with their quality of life can use advance directives to ensure that they will be resuscitated (see do not resuscitate orders, below). Issues related to the subjects of the value of life and quality of life will be considered in a Chapter 6 (p. 109).

The essential problem with advance directives is their ambiguity. Many patients take great pains to list all the types of care and treatment they will accept or reject under certain circumstances. Unfortunately, it is impossible to anticipate all the possible events that might make an advance directive necessary. No one can tell what their own death will be like and no one can anticipate how they will feel about their circumstances at the time. From a psychological perspective, we know that people change their attitudes and beliefs about things as they grow. Therefore, it would be wrong to assume that I can make a choice for myself at present that will be consistent with my attitudes and beliefs 10 years from now, or even 10 minutes from now. In some senses, my life can change so radically that I might even say about myself that I am no longer the same person I was at the time I made the initial decision. Is it right for one person to make a decision for another person (even if, physically, these are the same person), especially one so important as refusing treatment that will probably lead to death? This perspective might seem a bit far-fetched, as our intuitions will lead us to believe that we are somehow continuous and ought to have a right to make decisions about our futures even if we are not prepared to accept the eventual consequences. To protect people who change their minds, individuals are free to accept or reject their advance directives whenever they choose. One disturbing problem remains for advance directives: what if I change my mind but am not in a position to let anyone else know?

It is these sorts of ambiguities that cause us to be cautious about the supposed benefits of advance directives. Family members and doctors will eventually be left to construct relevant interpretations of the instructions left by patients. As a result, healthcare professionals should accept advance directives only after thoughtful discussion with the patient as to their anticipated wishes, fears and ideals.

Physician-assisted suicide (PAS)

There is wide debate over who is the most appropriate person to perform euthanasia. Patients like James Brady, who are unable to end their own lives, are at the mercy of those who might assist them, but less disabled patients could still prefer to seek assistance to ensure they receive the painless and dignified deaths they desire. Assisted suicide is described as:

> Assisting another person to end his or her life at that person's express wish. The legal definition of what constitutes 'assisting' varies from country to country.'[12]

There are sound arguments for insisting that doctors are the least appropriate to assist in suicide because '...it would contravene professional oaths and codes of ethics...; it would damage the relationship between doctors and patients...' and could lead to 'morally objectionable forms of euthanasia, such as involuntary euthanasia for the disabled'.[13] Others argue that doctors are most appropriate to assist in this way because they have a suitable educational background and skill.[14]

PAS is usually associated with active euthanasia, such as lethal injections to intentionally terminate a life. Certain forms of passive euthanasia are more likely to be accepted by the medical profession. Institutions tend to use mechanisms and policies for ratifying passive forms of euthanasia, such as non-resuscitation of dying or severely incapacitated patients.

At present it is illegal for a doctor in the UK to assist in a suicide. Nevertheless, all doctors ought to consider how they would react if a patient or loved one asked them for help to die.

Do not resuscitate orders (DNROs)

These are statements, which can be included in a patient's notes, saying that the patient has consented to not being resuscitated. They are a form of institutionally recognized advance directive, usually supported by healthcare workers, patients and the law.

Although they look like medical decisions, it must be very clear that DNROs are decided on the basis of value judgements. It is always the case that the DNRO is issued because the quality of life of the patient is believed to be so diminished that it is no longer desirable. This can sound harsh out of context, but the family of Janet Johnstone, for example, might have found it a welcome, though regrettable, release. However, people with disabilities have been alarmed by the recent move by the British Medical Association towards a policy on DNROs. They feel strongly that their lives could be deemed of too low quality to merit resuscitation by doctors who make the decision without enough insight. Thus, it is best if the patient gives proper informed consent to the order.

Matters are complicated when patients refuse the DNRO and it is clear that their condition will be considerably worse if they are resuscitated, such as very infirm patients. In such a case, two principles clash. Patient autonomy should be respected, although doctors do not have to perform a treatment that is perceived to be futile and burdensome. However, it is important to consider that the value perspectives of the practitioner might differ from those of the patient. Hence, DNROs are most appropriately used with informed consent from the patient.

Arguments for and against euthanasia

Finally, we come to consideration of the correctness of euthanasia. Arguments in favour of euthanasia usually take the form of arguments for the right to die. This is a right that suggests that:

> Some individuals, whose decisions for suicide plainly cannot be dismissed as irrational or foolish or premature, must be accorded a reasonable opportunity to show that their decision for death is informed and free… [Otherwise, it would mean that a] citizen does not, after all, have the right, even in principle, to live and die in the light of his own religious and ethical beliefs, his own convictions about why his life is valuable and where its value lies.[15]

The claim here is that euthanasia is a right to die that affirms the desires and values of the person who requests it. Other proponents claim that euthanasia is the most merciful response to certain kinds of suffering.

Opponents tend to be concerned about the voluntariness of euthanasia. They claim that many patients would submit under duress if they felt pressured to die rather than be burdens on their families. This concern frequently belies a further concern that general support of euthanasia could lead down a slippery slope toward involuntary active euthanasia. They fear that once we accept *some* forms of euthanasia there is little to stop us from accepting *any* form of euthanasia. This position could be unjustified given that so far all bills in favour of euthanasia are restricted to certain types and demand strong legal restrictions to guard against such possibilities. In fact, proponents and opponents alike argue in favour of strict legislation to guard against the slippery slope.

Other arguments against euthanasia are based on a tension between the quality of life and the sanctity of life. These two perspectives will be considered in greater detail in Chapter 6. In this context, the arguments emphasize that any life is valuable as a life, and is worth living regardless of its perceived quality. The sanctity of life position is rejected by proponents of the right to die on the grounds that people of sound mind must have the right to judge the quality of their own lives and consequently what value their lives have to them.

Palliative care[16]

Despite some people's strong convictions, a patient's desire to die does not necessarily imply a duty on the doctor's part to assist the patient in a suicide. The law and professional bodies certainly do not accept assisted suicide as an appropriate activity for a doctor, and consider it criminal behaviour even if the circumstances mitigate in its favour. Still, many patients will be in pain and distress at the end of their lives; some will seek help in the form of assisted suicide, others just want help to alleviate their distress. Alternatives must be available for patients requesting euthanasia and for patients who require care that is not intended to be curative. Palliative care offers a means of coping with the pain and indignity of terminal illness and long-term debilitating conditions.

There is a significant difference between extending life and prolonging a death that may be painful and undignified. Palliative care attempts to bridge the gap between these possibilities by adding a third option, one that seeks neither to extend life *where it would be futile* and is no longer possible to do so, nor to prolong the suffering and anguish of a painful and undignified death. The palliative option includes pain relief and brings independence and dignity to the process of dying. It releases the patient from futile attempts at extending life and thereby avoids unnecessary prolongation of death.

Cure versus care

It is worth considering that there is a legitimate difference between treatment that is curative and care for the patient. Palliative medicine is founded on the principle that something can be done even when cure is no longer probable. Thus care is considered to be management aimed at restoring function, dignity and independence even when it is no longer possible to extend the patient's life. This approach prizes quality over quantity when all else has failed. No case is considered hopeless because we are never helpless to do something for the patient. It demonstrates that patients who cannot be restored to full health need not be ignored by their caregivers, because good quality of life is still achievable in many cases. Elizabeth Stenhouse, a therapy radiographer, wrote on this topic: 'the dying have a right to be treated as whole people with living still to be done' (personal communication).

Practitioners will be reassured to know that, in most cases, something can be done for a patient, even if cure is unlikely. This is significant because the upshot of failing to recognize that something can be done often causes misperceptions that lead to misplaced blame for our frustrations. In situations where the patient is dying despite our best efforts, frustration can lead to the patient being labelled difficult and being ignored by doctors who blame themselves because they feel they have nothing left to give. If doctors realize they can help by providing pain relief, care and assistance, they will feel empowered and be less likely see the situation as a failure for which they blame the patient or are afraid to confront the patient. Doctors are still needed in the dying context. The need for care remains the same, but the type of care changes in end of life or non-curative situations. Consider the following real-life case.

Case 21
Ol' Joe

Ol' Joe was a 68-year-old male patient in a long-term care hospital attached to a retirement home. He had been living in the hospital for at least 3 years, and was well liked by the staff. Joe was admitted with a heavy drinking habit but worked hard to cut down, with the help of the staff. However, he subsequently developed a dependency on painkillers prescribed for an arthritic knee. Once again, the staff worked hard to help wean Joe from the medication. He lived quite contentedly in the hospital for a few years, although the staff were always wary of prescribing addictive medications for him. Joe usually cooperated with this decision, sometimes forfeiting adequate pain control to avoid further addiction.

One morning, Joe complained he was in pain and couldn't walk when an orderly tried to help him out of bed. At first, the staff assumed that he was looking for attention and drugs; however, the same thing happened on three successive mornings, so a doctor was called in. Within a few days, tests revealed that Joe was suffering from advanced prostate cancer, which was what was causing the pain in his back and legs. The cancer was incurable and the staff were saddened by their friend's illness. Nevertheless, they were reluctant to give him morphine-related drugs because of his history of substance abuse, and when Joe complained he was treated as if he was engaging in his addictive behaviour again.

The significant element of the case for the purposes of this section is the reluctance of the staff to prescribe opiates to control the patient's pain. It is among the first considerations in care that patients be given help without causing unnecessary harm. In this case, the staff made their decision not to prescribe opiates because of their previous knowledge of Joe's addictive behaviour. They expressed concern that they would be harming Joe by putting him in a situation where he would likely have to undergo the suffering of withdrawal if he became addicted again.

Addictions have serious consequences for those who live with them. People who are addicted to certain substances are frequently described as living with diminished autonomy because the addiction affects their ability to make free and rational choices. Addiction restricts the addicted person's priorities, causing them to make decisions just to maintain the addiction. Addicts will be hindered from acting freely because their reason for action will always be affected by their need to acquire and use the substance to

which they are addicted. Therefore, addiction is considered harmful not simply because the addictive substances can have unhealthy or destructive side effects but also because it diminishes autonomy. It is therefore reasonable for the staff to feel they would be causing Joe harm if they offered him potentially addictive medication that he would need to be weaned from in the long term. This is consistent with a deontological duty not to harm patients. It is also consistent with consequentialism, as the long term outcomes of addiction can justify short-term harm of living with greater pain.

This notwithstanding, it is not likely that Joe was going to survive long enough to become addicted or to need withdrawal. In the case study, Joe is dying because of the cancer, even if his death was not imminent. The staff's concerns about potential addiction were therefore unnecessary and unfounded because they were irrelevant to Joe. Instead, the staff should have been considering which alternatives were most suitable to someone suffering from the end stages of cancer.

The context of the case is relevant here. Staff members in long-term care hospital have experiences that impact on their values and perceptions of care and patients. This set of healthcare practitioners was engaged in care of the elderly and infirm, most of whom were dying but many of whose deaths were not imminent. Joe had been in the hospital for years before he began to die from cancer. This means the care team was geared towards assisting patients to live with as much independence as possible, not towards helping them die. It was therefore difficult for them to change gear and to recognize that the management plan that had suited Joe before he developed cancer was no longer suitable when the cancer began to kill him. The case demonstrates how values and expectations can interfere with care. The solution is to be open to the possibility of change and recognition that the values of long-term medicine are not all relevant in the palliative context.

In the end, Joe received the kind of care and assistance he required because the team gathered for a discussion of the case with a an external observer who simply asked 'Is this patient dying?' All the staff were relieved to have reassessed the reality of the situation, which permitted them to provide the patient with some kind of care even if it was not the kind they were used to giving him. He died a few weeks later, but his pain and his relationship with the staff had improved. Death in this case was not a failure but a regrettable necessity. The success was in ensuring that he died in comfort and with dignity. In addition, the staff felt empowered to do something for him.

More often, similar dilemmas arise in situations where a treatment is available but the patient's illness is so far advanced that cure is no longer probable and death is likely. In such cases, the elements of utility and futility become relevant, as discussed above. As we have seen, there is no duty for doctors to offer futile therapy even if the options are available; there is no duty to treat the untreatable. Doing so can cause harm by unnecessarily prolonging death. Nevertheless, there is no reason for patients to die with unnecessary suffering and this is where palliation comes in. Not curing does not imply ignoring the patient. A lot can be done to help the patient to die with dignity and limited suffering.

Sedation into unconsciousness

A further dilemma related to death and dying is whether and when it is appropriate to sedate a patient into unconsciousness. It is possible that patients might suffer so greatly either from physical or emotional pain near the end of their lives that nothing can be done to relieve them. Given the moral and legal restrictions against assisted

suicide, it might be tempting to help patients by keeping them unconscious and unaware of their condition. It is debatable whether this is a legitimate solution for suffering patients. To some it will be a welcome relief, to others a fate worse than death to remain alive but incapable of experience or participation in life. Similarly, to some, life in advanced stages of dementia or in persistent vegetative state is of such diminished quality that it is not worth living. To others the mere presence of life is valuable at any cost. This is a matter of conscience for each of us to determine. It is an issue that will be discussed in Chapter 6.

Organ donation, transplantation and xenotransplantation

The chief problem associated with organ transplantation is the scarcity of organs available for donation. From this core resource problem flow virtually all other ethical problems associated with organ donation and transplantation. The ethical debate about distributive justice and resource allocation is covered in depth in Chapter 9. The arguments considered there are relevant to most of what will be said in this section, so the two ought to be considered together. However, there is no doubt that organ donation and transplantation is a life and death subject, and so it will be covered among the ethical concerns about death and dying.

The shortage of organs

There are patients all over the world on waiting lists to receive organ transplants. In some cases these will be life-saving to those who receive them, in other cases they will restore a quality of life believed vital by the individual concerned. There is a shortage of organs available and the result is competition, disappointment and tragic situations where people die before they reach the top of the waiting list. How can this situation be resolved?

In the UK, the Human Organs Transplant Act (1989) was enacted to oversee the appropriate cultivation, use and distribution of organs for transplantation. This Act resulted from a scandal in the late 1980s in which doctors had been discovered to be buying organs from living people. These were usually single kidneys bought from healthy individuals who could survive very well with the one remaining kidney. However, the recognition that poor people, mostly immigrants, were being paid to donate vital organs scandalized the nation with concerns about exploitation of people desperate for money to support themselves and their families.[17]

The consensus seems to be that the buying and selling of human organs for transplantation is exploitative and unacceptable. This embodies values of respect for bodily integrity and non-maleficence, but could interfere with autonomy. Should individuals have the right to sell their organs if they so choose? The assumption is that only people in desperate and oppressed situations will choose to do so and it is not clear that they will be acting freely if they do. Desperation implies a form of coercion in which the individual will resort to degrading means to accomplish their ends, leaving open the likelihood of exploitation.[18]

However, the act does not interfere with the autonomous right to donate organs. Under this light, tissue and organs have been donated to family members, and even strangers, because it was possible to do so and not because it was financially rewarding.

Even despite the possibility of generous gifts, waiting lists continue to grow and people fail to receive organs that will save their lives. How can the imbalance be rectified? Many options have been made available and drastic measures have been put into place to attempt to relieve the pressure on waiting lists. In the UK, people are invited to sign organ donor cards that will act as advance directives, permitting the removal of their organs for transplantation in the event of their death. This is a popular model employed in many countries. It is consistent with respect for autonomy because it permits people to make their own choice about the issue and to make their decision known. It also preserves a very valuable asset of society, namely the ability to act in a charitable way. Organ donation is arguably a very generous gift that will be greatly appreciated by its recipient. However, it can also be argued that the gift, after death, is rather small, given that the donor will no longer benefit from the organ. Still, it is important to consider whether removing the freedom to give in this way would somehow diminish us socially by removing an overt act of generosity.

This should not be an issue, as no one will prevent another person from donating their organs after death unless they are unusable for clinical reasons. So how could charity be lost? Charity would be a casualty of removing the right to opt in or contract into donation by signing an organ donor card by choice; and indeed, the reverse has been proposed. This is often called the opting-out or contracting-out alternative. In this case, people would be asked to sign a card if they did *not* wish their organs procured for transplantation. Otherwise it would be presumed upon death that all individuals who have not contracted out agree to have their organs removed for the purposes of donation. The opting-out policy has been tried in countries such as Belgium, to great apparent success. The waiting list for organs greatly reduced after the contracting-out law was passed and thousands of people have benefited so far. And yet, people are still upset by the proposal that their organs will be harvested by presumption of consent as opposed to clear overt consent. The concern is for people who forget to sign their cards, but more important is the implication that opting out entails

– that one's body becomes the possession of the state after death until it has been used for donation. Is this a fair assumption? Or could it be that contracting-out simply makes more sense than relying on individuals to remember to find and fill in a form?

A compromise position might be possible. In New Zealand, for example, people must complete organ donation cards if they want a driver's licence. This means that a large proportion of the population has to think about and either donate or refuse to donate their organs before they are permitted to drive. As more people are concerned about having a driver's licence than choosing to opt in or out of an organ donation scheme, the method manages to include a high number of people who might never think about the issues and never get around to filling in a card.

> Think about the advantages and disadvantages of these options.

In the end, a policy on organ donation and procurement will have to consider if donation is a duty or an act of charity. If it becomes a duty then it benefits by being of greater use to those who require organ donations for survival, but this will diminish opportunities for acts of generosity. On the other hand, depending on acts of charity based on contracting-in policies has brought us no nearer to helping all those who could be helped.

Currently, doctors must ask permission from relatives to harvest organs from the deceased. This is a sensitive and difficult request that many people would prefer to avoid. It is hard to ask mourning relatives such a question just as they are having to cope with the news of the death of a loved one. However, it might be reassuring to the relatives to know that someone will be helped from the death, knowledge that could add value to the death and richness to the life lost. The request must be handled

sensitively, and communication skills classes can help by giving pointers and, more importantly, using role-play for practice. However, we cannot ignore the moral responsibility to ask because it could be the only chance for an anxious recipient waiting for a life-saving transplant.

Families are usually prepared to consent or refuse consent for organs to be harvested if they know of the patient's wishes in that area. However, it is generally accepted that families are permitted to refuse to consent. Is this right, considering the number of people who are waiting for transplantations? Refusal can always be justified if it is not clear what the patient would have wished, i.e. if no directive was given in advance. Families are therefore consulted on the presumption that they will know the patient's wishes in this respect. Moreover, it is the family that is suffering the bereavement and it is thought to be respectful to ask them to decide what will be done with the body. Signing a donor card will make a person's choice clear to their family members and will prepare them in advance for this question.

Who will receive and how is this determined

The recognition that organs are not readily available raises a significant question about who will receive organs when they do become available and how these decisions will be made.

Case 22
Who will live?

In April 1997, allegations were made against a Scottish transplant unit that a 15-year-old girl was refused a liver transplant because, as her grandmother put it 'we just weren't worth bothering with'. Michelle, the girl, died of liver failure related to recreational drug use. The hospital claimed that it had refused the operation on moral grounds, presumably related to the discovery that Michelle had used

> cannabis against her doctor's warning, while she was in hospital for treatment. The grandmother's concern was that Michelle was being discriminated against because she had abused drugs and her mother was a recovering drug addict. However, as she and her lawyer pointed out, that same week a well-known football player with a history of alcoholism was given a second liver transplant at the same hospital.[19]

This sad and emotive case, which attracted considerable media attention, was the subject of a Fatal Accident Injury (see p. 79). In his written determination the Sheriff indicated that the fact this girl used recreational drugs played no part in the decisions made by doctors about her management and the decision not to carry out a transplant. However this case raises the issue of whether social criteria should impose themselves on decisions such as this.

Some suggest that an individual's past social behaviour can be used as an indicator of how likely they are to be able to cope with the strict regimen and abstinence required after a transplant operation. Others point out that this approach simply serves to select patients with a similar set of values and worldviews as the decision makers.

When there are not enough organs to go round is it possible to discriminate between possible recipients? Are some people more 'deserving' than others for either past achievements or future promise? Are others less 'derserving' because of their behaviour? Perhaps we should concern ourselves with maximising the associated benefits for the patients' families, dependents and friends.

In some cases, the media favour particular patients and pressure the choice. In at least one case, the family of a newborn child with heart defect appeared on a talk-show and was given an immediate donation after a couple mourning the death of their own child heard their plea. Baby Jesse had been refused a transplant and his family charged that the decision was made on social grounds because of the instability of the parents' background. After the television appearance, Baby Jesse jumped the queue, receiving a transplant ahead of all other babies waiting at the time. Two obvious value judgements were made, one that placed Baby Jesse at the end of the queue and one that moved him to the head.[20] They prove that there is some reason for concern about the way that such decisions are made and the application of value judgements to the process.

Rank the following patients for a life-saving heart transplant:

1. A 37-year-old mother of three children who has never smoked and rarely drinks alcohol
2. 23-year-old civil servant and former Olympics hopeful
3. A Gulf War veteran with medals for acts of bravery
4. A former alcoholic who now counsels families of alcoholics
5. A 62-year-old heart surgeon
6. A 54-year-old schoolteacher who used to smoke two packs of cigarettes a day.

What criteria did you use?

Live donation and gifts

Not all organ recipients rely on deceased donors. Some donors are living and can donate, for example, bone marrow, blood or kidneys. Where a family member or friend is concerned about the prospects of a particular individual it is possible for them to arrange a gift donation, and frequently that is the first place a donation will be sought. This is usually for clinical reasons, because there is a greater chance of success between family members. However, two recent occurrences have raised ethical dilemmas regarding live donation.

The father who wanted to give too much?
In one case, a father wanted to donate his one remaining kidney to his son. He had already donated a kidney to his younger son, but both young men had inherited the same congenital disorder from their mother and the second son was now in need of a transplant. Should the father be permitted to donate his one remaining kidney? Many were not convinced it would be a good idea for him to make the sacrifice, but he was willing. Others thought it was just a way of creating a new patient, because the father would then depend on dialysis for his survival. He was prepared to live with this because he felt he had had a fair chance in life and his son had not. Should the father be allowed to donate his kidney and create his own ill health? What if he should require a kidney transplant in the future? Would he be entitled to it, having given up his kidney? Would he have earned it by his good deed? A deontologist would probably praise the father for his generosity and sense of duty towards his family. A utilitarian might condemn him for adding to the burden on the health budget.

Refusal to provide donation
A second dilemma regards potential donors who refuse to donate. To protect people from consenting to donation by coercion it is necessary to permit a refusal to take part. This relieves anyone from pressure to consent and also protects children from being consented for by parents. However, it is possible that a family member will refuse to make a life-saving donation and this raises moral problems.[21] We protect bodily integrity by not forcing people to submit to donation but, in cases where a life could be saved by the donation, this is difficult to condone. Ultimately, we protect the individual right to autonomy and bodily integrity, even at the expense of life. It would be hard to justify any other possibility. There is more discussion of the notion of bodily integrity in Chapter 8.

Some people refuse to sign their organ donor cards because of fears of elective ventilation, and this is a problem the law has taken very seriously. At present, it is illegal in the UK to keep a body in a living state for more than a few minutes. This means that it is not permissible to apply elective ventilation for the purposes of harvesting organs. Respect for bodily integrity is cited here, but also respect of the family of the deceased, who ought not to be expected to wait indefinitely for the body to be released for burial. Is this acceptable?

Xenotransplantation and cloning

A relatively new alternative to organ donation between humans is xenotransplantation – transplantation across species. Pigs and baboons have been used experimentally for transplant and it will not be long before the technology is advanced enough to make it readily available. Many objections have surfaced over the use of animals for these purposes. It has been deemed exploitative, although it is difficult to condemn in a society that relies on meat for nourishment. The main concern is the potential danger to the community of transgenic animals producing retroviruses that could affect entire populations. Animals would need to have their genes transformed to make them more compatible to the human recipients. This transgenesis could lead to changes in viruses that are currently only mild or harmless in humans. HIV is believed to be such a retrovirus. The claim is that introducing such a virus to animal–human genetic mutations could generate an infectious disease, more virulent and uncontrollable than HIV, with the wide-ranging and debilitating effects of bubonic plague. To safeguard against this, a moratorium was placed on xenotransplantation and recipients will have to agree to certain restrictions, such as never to produce offspring (in whom the transgenesis will have unknown effects).[22]

Perhaps a safer option is one currently in development – the production of cloned organs for transplantation. People who needed new organs could give a sample of DNA from which the organ could be produced *in vitro*. So far, the technology to perform this is very distant, but it is not impossible. It would certainly help to relieve some of the ethical drawbacks associated with donation and xenotransplantation.

Fetal tissue implants are another concern, but these will be addressed in Chapter 8.

Conclusion

This chapter has focused on ethical issues related to death and dying. We have covered some of the emotive debate, using examples from real-life cases. Although the debate about euthanasia is ongoing, concepts have been clarified in an effort to assist those who must confront the realities of the debate in work and beyond. Ethical issues related to palliative care were discussed and the field was offered as an alternative to assisted suicide. Ethical challenges associated with organ donation and transplantation were analysed. It is up to individual practitioners to ensure they understand their duties related to end of life issues and consider how they wish to respond.

Notes and references

1 See: Gavaghan C. Voluntary Euthanasia Society of Scotland website. Available at: http://www.euthanasia.org/history.html See also: Mercy killing brother admonished. The Herald; 15 October 1996 and Man who killed incurable brother freed. The Guardian; 15 October 1996 and The courage to kill the one you love. The Observer; 27 October 1996.
2 Gavaghan C. VESS website. Available at: http://www.euthanasia.org/history.html
3 Boyd K et al. The new dictionary of medical ethics. London: British Medical Journal Publishing; 1997:76.
4 Gavaghan C. VESS website. Available at: http://www.euthanasia.org/history.html
5 Tumelty M. I will stay with my mum to the end. Daily Record; 25 April 1996.
6 Dyer C. Scottish court gives right to die. Br Med J 1996; 312:1115.
7 Dyer C. Scottish court gives right to die. Br Med J 1996; 312:1115.
8 British Medical Association. Withholding and withdrawing life-prolonging medical treatment: guidance for decision making. London: BMJ Books; 1999.
9 Submission from the Ethics Group of the Association of Palliative Medicine of Great Britain and Ireland to the Select Committee of the House of Lords on Medical Ethics. May 1996:6.
10 Street K et al. The decision-making process regarding the withdrawal or withholding of potential life-saving treatments in a children's hospital. J Medical Ethics 2000; 26:346–352.
11 Slowther A et al. Clinical ethics support services in the UK: an investigation of the current provision of ethics support to health professionals in the UK. J Medical Ethics 2001; 27:2i–8i.
12 See: the index and glossary of the Scottish Voluntary Euthanasia Society. Available at: http://www.euthanasia.org/a_z.html See also: Britton A, McLean S. First British research on assisted suicide announced. Available at: http://www.euthanasia.org/96-3mcln.html
13 Elliot C. Philosopher assisted suicide. Br Med J 1996; 313:1088–1089.
14 Dworkin R et al. Assisted suicide: the philosopher's brief. New York Review of Books; 1997. Available from On-line Archives: http://www.nybooks.com:6900/nyrev/WWWfeatdisplay.cgi?1997032741F@p1
15 Dworkin R et al. Assisted suicide: the philosopher's brief. New York Review of Books; 1997. Available from On-line Archives: http://www.nybooks.com:6900/nyrev/WWWfeatdisplay.cgi?1997032741F@p1
16 Randall F, Downie RS. Palliative care ethics: a good companion. Oxford: Oxford University Press; 1996.
17 Turks had 'compelling' reasons to sell organs. The Independent. April 1990.
18 Nuffield Council on Bioethics. Human tissues: ethical and legal issues. Available at: http@//www.nuffield.org/bioethics/publication/humantissue/rep0013057.html
19 Riddell P. Baxter had two liver ops, Michelle died because she never got one. The Sun; 29 April 1997:7.
20 For a detailed treatment of this case, see Thomas J, Waluchow W. Well and good: case studies in biomedical ethics. Peterborough, Ontario: Broadview Press; 1990.
21 In the US, the court refused to force a donation in the case of *McFall* v. *Schimp* (1978).
22 Nuffield Council on Bioethics. Animal to human transplants: the ethics of xenotransplantation. Available at: http://www.nuffield.org/bioethics/publication/transplants/rep0011258.html

6

The value of life: who decides and how?

Questions about the value of life involve some of the most important considerations made in the fields of medicine and medical ethics, including treatment and management decisions in all areas of life and death. Placing a value on a given life is significant in antenatal care, infant care, childhood, adulthood and into old age. It is relevant to congenital birth defects and genetic conditions, as well as to mid-life accidents and senile dementia. How we make decisions regarding the value of a given life, and who ought to make these decisions, is difficult to discern (Fig. 6.1). Perhaps most importantly of all, why are we even interested in assessing the value of a life?

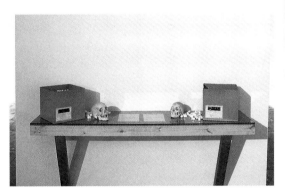

Figure 6.1
The title of this installation piece – '2nd class male, 2nd class female' – raises the question of whether it is ever appropriate to place a value on life. The company that sold these skulls for educational purposes had labelled them 'second class' because they were considered to be of poor educational quality. ('2nd class male, 2nd class female' Christine Borland 1996. © Christine Borland. Courtesy of the artist and Howard and Donna Stone, Chicago.)

Consider the following case.

Case 23
The value of life

Katherine Lewis is an intelligent, unmarried, 40-year-old woman suffering from Guillain–Barré's syndrome, a painful neurological illness that leaves its sufferers paralysed for unpredictable lengths of time. Many people recover from the syndrome more or less completely and live long, relatively healthy lives. However, Katherine has been paralysed for 3 years and, 10 months ago, it was recognized that she was unlikely to be able to move or breathe on her own again because of the extent of damage to her nerves and muscles; she now needs a ventilator to help her breathe.

You explained this to Katherine in a gentle but clear manner. Last week Katherine asked to speak with you privately. She told you that she had considered her options and decided that she no longer wanted to live. She said her life held no value for her if it meant being in constant pain and without the freedom to move or even breathe on her own. She told you that she has discussed this with her family and that they have accepted her wishes to have the ventilator removed.

The case illustrates the relevance of questioning the value of a life, if for no other reason than that some people come face-to-face with the reality of asking this question about their own lives. The key consideration in end of life challenges is how that life is valued. In the case of James Brady (see p. 91), it became clear that Brady placed little value on his life as his health began to fail. On balance, he preferred to die rather than continue to live with the quality to which his life had deteriorated. The courts made the same decision for Janet Johnstone after recommendations from her family and doctors (see p. 96). Similarly, Katherine Lewis, in the case above, made a long-considered decision about the value of her own life. So the issue is relevant. Nevertheless, how the value of a life is determined is so far unanswerable, although there are some useful ideas and principles to consider.

In this section we will consider first *how* decisions about the value of life are made and, second, *who* is, and ought to be, involved in these decisions. The first question will be resolved by exploring concepts of quality, quantity and sanctity of life. We will also examine the differences involved when making decisions about individual lives as distinct from making general decisions about the value of types of lives (in other words, we will distinguish decisions made at the micro and macro levels). The second aspect will explore the differences between stakeholders and decision makers, and ask who has a legitimate stake in the decisions about value of life and who ought to be permitted to make those decisions. We will ask:

- how do we place value on life?
- who are the relevant stakeholders and decision-makers?

How do we place value on life?

There are essentially three elements to consider when determining the value of life:

- quality
- quantity
- sanctity.

Quality

The first criterion that springs to mind regarding the value of life is usually the quality of the life or lives in question:

> The quality of life ethic puts the emphasis on the type of life being lived, not upon the fact of life. Lives are not all of one kind; some lives are of great value to the person himself and to others while others are not. What the life means to someone is what is important. Keeping this in mind it is not inappropriate to say that some lives are of greater value than others, that the condition or meaning of life does have much to do with the justification for terminating that life.[1]

Those who choose to reason on this basis hope that if the quality of a life can be measured then the answer to whether that life has value to the individual can be determined easily. This raises special problems, however, because the idea of quality involves a value judgement, and value judgements are, by their essence, subject to indeterminate relative factors such as preferences and dislikes. Hence, quality of life is difficult to measure and will vary according to individual tastes, preferences and aspirations. As a result, no general rules or principles can be asserted that would simplify decisions about the value of a life based on its quality. Nevertheless, quality is still an essential criterion in making such decisions because it gives legitimacy to the possibility that rational, autonomous persons can decide for themselves that their own lives either are worth, or are no longer worth, living. To disregard this possibility would be to imply that no individuals can legitimately make such value judgements about their own lives and, if nothing else, that would be counterintuitive.[2] In our case, Katherine Lewis had spent 10 months considering her decision before concluding that her life was no longer of a tolerable quality. She put a great deal of effort into the decision and she was competent when she made it. Who would be better placed to make this judgement for her than Katherine herself? And yet, a doctor faced with her request would most likely be uncertain about whether Katherine's choice is truly in her best interest, and feel trepidation about assisting her. We need to know which considerations can be used to protect the patient's interests.

> Write a list of three things that make your life worth living and ask someone else to do the same.
>
> Compare your lists.
>
> Are they identical? Why?
>
> Are they not identical? Why not?

The quality of life criterion asserts that there is a difference between the *type* of life and the *fact* of life. This is the primary difference between it and the sanctity criterion discussed on page 115. Among quality of life considerations rest three assertions:

1. there is relative value to life
2. the value of a life is determined subjectively
3. not all lives are of equal value.

Relative value
The first assertion, that life is of relative value, could be taken in two ways. In one sense, it could mean that the value of a given life can be placed on a scale and measured against other lives. The scale could be a social scale, for example, where the contributions or potential for contribution of individuals are measured against those of fellow citizens. Critics of quality of life criteria frequently name this as a potential slippery slope where lives would be deemed worthy of saving, or even not saving, based on the relative social value of the individual concerned. So, for example, a mother of four children who is a practising doctor could be regarded of greater value to the community than an unmarried accountant. The concern is that the potential for discrimination is too high.

Because of the possibility of prejudice and injustice, supporters of the quality of life criterion reject this interpersonal construction in favour of a second, more personalized, option. According to this interpretation, the notion of relative value is relevant not between individuals but within the context of one person's life and is measured against that person's needs and aspirations. So Katherine would base her decision on a comparison between her life before and after her illness. The value placed on the quality of a life would be determined by the individual depending on whether he or she believes the current state to be relatively preferable to previous or future states and whether he or she can foresee controlling the circumstances that make it that way. Thus, the life of an athlete who aspires to participate in the Olympics can be changed in relative value by an accident that leaves that person a quadriplegic. The athlete might decide that the relative value of her life is diminished after the accident, because she perceives her desires and aspirations to be reduced or beyond her capacity to control. However, if she receives treatment and counselling her aspirations could change and, with the adjustment, she could learn to value her life as a quadriplegic as much or more than her previous life. This illustrates how it is possible for a person to adjust the values by which they appraise their lives. For Katherine Lewis, the decision went the opposite way and she decided that a life of incapacity and constant pain was of relatively low value to *her*.

It is not surprising that the most vociferous protesters against permitting people in Katherine's position to be assisted in terminating their lives are people who themselves are disabled. Organizations run by, and that represent, persons with disabilities make two assertions in this light. First, they claim that accepting that Katherine Lewis has a right to die based on her determination that her life is of relatively little value is demeaning to all disabled people, and implies that any life with a severe disability is not worth living. Their second assertion is that with proper help, over time Katherine would be able to transform her personal outlook and find satisfaction in her life that would increase its relative value for her.

The first assertion can be addressed by clarifying that the case of Katherine Lewis must not be taken as a general rule. Deontologists, who are interested in knowing general principles and duties that can be applied across all cases would not be very satisfied with this; they would prefer to be able to look to duties that would apply in all cases. Here, a case-based, context-sensitive approach is better suited. Contextualizing would permit freedom to act within a particular context, without the implication that the decision must hold in general. So, in this case, Katherine might decide that her life is relatively valueless. In another case, for example that of actor Christopher Reeve, the decision to seek other ways of valuing this major life change led to him perceiving his life as highly valuable, even if different in value from before the accident that made him a paraplegic. This invokes the second assertion, that Katherine could change her view over time. Although we recognize this is possible in some cases, it is not clear how it applies to Katherine. Here we have a case in which a rational and competent person has had time to consider her options and has chosen to end her life of suffering beyond what she believes she can endure. Ten months is a long time and it will have given her plenty of opportunity to consult with family and professionals about the possibilities open to her in the future. Given all this, it is reasonable to assume that Katherine has made a well-reasoned decision. It might not be a decision that everyone can agree with but if her reasoning process can be called into question then at what point can we say that a decision is sound? She meets all the criteria for competence and she is aware of the consequences of her decision. It would be very difficult to determine what arguments could truly justify interfering with her choice.

Subjective determination
The second assertion made by supporters of the quality of life as a criterion for decision-making is closely related to the first, but with an added dimension. This assertion suggests that the determination of the value of the quality of a given life is a subjective determination to be made by the person experiencing that life. The important addition here is that the decision is a personal one that, ideally, ought not to be made externally by another person but internally by the individual involved. Katherine Lewis made this decision for herself based on a comparison between two stages of her life. So did James Brady. Without this element, decisions based on quality of life criteria lack salient information and the patients concerned cannot give informed consent. Patients must be given the opportunity to decide for themselves whether they think their lives are worth living or not. To ignore or overlook patients' judgement in this matter is to violate their autonomy and their freedom to decide for themselves on the basis of relevant information about their future, and comparative consideration of their past. As the deontological position puts it so well, to do so is to violate the imperative that we must treat persons as rational and as ends in themselves.

It is important to remember the subjectivity assertion in this context, so as to emphasize that the judgement made about the value of a life ought to be made only by the person concerned and not by others. Of course, this presumes that the person deciding is conscious and competent to make the decision at all, which is especially complicated in cases when the patient is unconscious, immature or suffering from a mental illness, such as depression, that could distort their decision-making abilities. Thus, seeking patient choice is not always a viable option. Not all patients are capable of choosing for themselves. In Janet Johnstone's case, and in the similar case of Tony Bland, the decision was made externally, by people involved in their care. In such situations, family or practitioners have been known to make the decision on behalf of the incompetent patient, usually because they claim to know what the patient in question would have wanted. Relatives and doctors of Janet Johnstone argued that her condition lacked the dignity and control she valued, and that her situation would not improve. Under the circumstances, the judge decided the quality of her life was so diminished that her life was no longer worth living and that Ms Johnstone herself would have reached the same conclusion.

The same sort of proxy decision making occurs when a woman, or couple, decide to terminate a pregnancy based on antenatal screening and testing. Here, parents make the decision on behalf of a fetus or a child.

Case 24
Screening/testing for Down syndrome

A 42-year-old woman presented at an antenatal clinic with her husband to discuss the results of her recent amniocentesis. In addition to Down syndrome, echocardiography of the fetus showed cardiac abnormalities, including atrioventricular septal defect. After extensive discussion between the parents and the obstetrician, the parents decided that the fetus had too many problems and that it would be unfair to the unborn child and to their other four children to continue with the pregnancy.

In such cases the parents must decide if, on balance, their child's life is worth living given the possibility of pain and suffering or such inhibited interaction with the world that it would be of no value to the person living it. Needless to say, this is a difficult and trying dilemma for anyone to face. It also introduces a concern that underlies all prenatal screening programmes, in that these are supported by the social values implied by screening, which direct women towards termination of positive tested pregnancies.[3] In the past, women were barred from screening and testing for similar conditions if they had previously decided that they would not terminate a pregnancy if the fetus carried the genetic condition. Hence screening was meant to be followed by testing, and positive results were meant to be followed by termination of pregnancy. The conclusion this yields, like it or not, is that our screening programmes carry with them an implication that the lives of those who are affected with certain conditions ought to be terminated because they are of comparatively less value than the lives of those who are not. This is supported in law by Wrongful Life suits in which parents of people born with screenable genetic conditions, such as spina bifida, have successfully sued doctors for the burden involved in caring for those born with such conditions.[4] The problems associated with screening will be discussed elsewhere in Chapter 8 (p. 146–147). They are significant here because they elucidate the third assertion made by supporters of quality of life considerations in the medical context.

Equal or unequal value?
The third assertion is that, as a result of subjective and relative determinations about the quality of a life, lives can be seen to be of unequal value. At the extreme, it follows that it is possible to describe a life as valueless, especially when it is compared with the value of a life that has greater quality. In the case of the unborn fetus affected by a debilitating inherited condition, the welfare of the parents and their other children can be invested with greater value than the potential good of a potential child born with a severe disability. This allows us to make relative judgements among or between lives of individuals or groups. This is especially useful in healthcare economics, where decisions about distribution of resources rely on comparative information of the effectiveness of treatments. In this way it can be determined that resources will be made available for treatments that are more effective at improving quality of life in

particular conditions and not where the
quality of life is not improved or so diminished that improvements are too small to
justify.

This point will be developed more fully in
the section on quality-adjusted life-years
(QALYs) and rationing in Chapter 9 (p. 163).
Here, it is important to point to the possibility of making comparative judgements based
on assessments of the quality of life and to
emphasize that such judgements can be used
to inform decisions about distributing and
rationalizing scarce resources. As a result,
there is a concern about quality of life decisions being made for others without their
participation, and about decisions imposed
without their consent. Both these concerns
are tempered by the second assertion of the
quality of life ethic. This states that value
must be personally assessed by the individual concerned, and imposed externally only
in extreme circumstances where patients are
unable to decide on their own behalf and
their wishes can be reasonably determined.
An advance directive can be highly useful in
the latter case. If a balance is made between
both subjective determination and comparative decisions, we can avoid classifying a life
as of comparatively low value where the
person possessing it does not agree.

Basing value of life decisions on quality of
life has strong advantages. It:

- *Is subjective:* takes seriously personal
  assessments made by individuals about the
  quality of their own lives
- *Is flexible:* recognizes the possibility that the
  subjectively determined value of one's life
  can change
- *Is comparative:* recognizes that the way one
  life is valued need not impose the identical
  value on a similar life condition
- *Permits rational suicide:* recognizes that one
  can legitimately assert the relatively low
  value of one's own life.

No one denies the importance of a good
quality of life, or one that is acceptable to the
person who has to live it. However, some
argue that it is not the sole criterion upon
which to base value of life decisions. These
people include considerations of quantity
and sanctity in their determination.

Quantity

The value of the quantity of a life should not
be underestimated. In the past, so much
emphasis was placed on the quality of life
lived that quantity was virtually forgotten.
More recently, attitudes have changed and
consideration is given to the possibility that
a long life of diminished quality could be as
highly valued as a short life of high quality.
In some senses the comparison seems
absurd, unless we consider cases in which
patients have refused complicated or ago-
nising treatments that they perceived would
exacerbate their suffering rather than extend
their lives. Other patients prefer to extend
their lives at any cost or risk to them
because they value their existence so much
that they will sacrifice quality in favour of
quantity. This indicates that quantity ought
not to be mistaken for quality and that prolonging a patient's life might be nothing
more than a burdensome and painful exten-
sion of suffering for them and their loved
ones. However tempting it is for doctors to
provide whatever care they are capable of
providing, there is a responsibility to ensure
that the treatments are actually useful to the
patient and not unnecessarily burdensome.
This means that a cost–benefit analysis can
be usefully applied to a care management
plan for an individual patient. The aim is to
determine the extent to which treatment will
be helpful and where the healing stops and
the burden begins.

Quantity might not be identical with
quality but, often, increased quantity in medicine can be equal to cure or control of
disease and hence does enhance quality of
life. The Compression of Morbidity principle
cited by Downie and Calman is useful for
guiding these decisions:

Compression of morbidity principle: the objective of increasing life-span should be associated at the same time with an increasing quality of life or reduction of disability.[5]

So, provided quality of life is maintained or enhanced, quantity is a positive factor in healthcare.

There is a sense in which quality of life judgements are made in a wider context and not just as they pertain to particular patients. Health economists have long tried to determine the appropriateness of costly treatments on the basis of their burdensomeness and effectiveness. The most famous of these is a system known as QALYs. QALYs stand for quality-adjusted life-years, and are a means of making comparisons between health states. Equally concerned with quantity and quality, QALYs can be applied to a 'relative health states' scale. The problem is that these scales are themselves value-laden. Such issues will be covered in Chapter 9, where the idea of QALYs will be discussed as they relate to rationing and distribution of resources. They are introduced here because they show how a model for decision making can include the notions of quality and quantity discussed in this chapter. QALYs help decide which healthcare needs will be met by identifying which yield:

- the greatest amount of good for
- the greatest amount of time for
- the greatest number of people.

However, this utilitarian approach also involves a degree of casuistry: patients' QALYs are assessed and decisions are made on the basis of how well a treatment worked for them. The treatment with the most acceptance can then be applied exclusively. But all patients are unique, so what works for many will not work for all individuals. This is the classic problem with inductive arguments where particulars are used to imply generals.

Sanctity

Supporters of the sanctity of life ethic dismiss considerations about quality and quantity because, they assert:

- all life is worth living under any condition because of
- the inherent value of life.

The upshot of the theory is that quality of life, although desirable, is irrelevant to assessing the value of a life because all life is inherently valuable. Many supporters of the sanctity of life criterion say this is true only of human life, but there are religious groups who claim sanctity extends to all life. Either way, the sanctity of life principle states that all human life is worthy of preservation and hence eliminates the justifiability of abortion, euthanasia and rational suicide and, at extremes, withdrawal of futile treatment:

> The sanctity of life ethic holds that every human life is intrinsically good, that no life is more valuable than another, that lives not fully developed (embryonic and fetal stages) and lives with no great potential (the suffering lives of the terminally ill or the pathetic lives of the severely handicapped) are still sacred. The condition of a life does not reduce its value or justify its termination.[6]

So, whereas to determine the value of a life on its quality asserts that there is a relevant difference between the *type* of life and the *fact* of life, this distinction is rejected by sanctity arguments as irrelevant.

The sanctity criterion tends to be associated with religious beliefs. The Judeo-Christian rationale is usually that lives are inherently valuable because they are gifts from God and not ours to end as we wish. In a sense, our lives are on loan to us and, as such, must be treated with respect. In Islam, the suffering associated with reduced quality of life is also considered a divine endowment and therefore ought to be borne without assistance, as the suffering is said to lead to enlightenment and divine reward.

However, religious arguments are not required to defend sanctity beliefs. It is enough simply to say that all human lives are deserving of equal respect not because of what they have to offer or have offered or potentially will offer, but because they exist. The notion of inalienable human rights attributes force to the value of human life with the assertion that it needs no justification. This is the primary merit of the sanctity of life ethic – that a life requires no justification – but justification *is* required for the premature termination of that life. In this sense, the principle acts as a forceful bulwark against devaluing human life. Article 3 of the United Nations Declaration of Human rights asserts simply that:

> Everyone has the right to life, liberty and security of person.[7]

No argument is made to justify this claim because no argument is necessary. However, it will be necessary to justify any violation of this right.

The sanctity of life criterion is appealing because it appears to resolve a number of ethical quandaries. To accept it would entail rejection of so many of the problematic issues faced by practitioners and ethicists. For instance, it will mean rejecting abortion at any stage of pregnancy because of the inherent value of the life of the fetus. This seems like an easy solution to the problem of abortion, except in cases where a pregnancy might be terminated to save the life of the mother. In such cases, sanctity of life cannot inform the decision of which life should be saved. On the one hand, we might choose to save the mother's life because she is already viable and independent and she might have responsibilities that give her life added value. On the other hand, we could save the fetus which, although only a potential life, has not had the opportunity to live that the mother has had, and so deserves a

chance. The list of reasons can be given on behalf of either life, but this is no solution. In fact, all it does is present us with reasons to use quality and quantity criteria for resolving the dilemma. This is a serious practical shortcoming of the sanctity criterion. Other problems will be discussed below.

Problems faced by the quality, quantity and sanctity criteria

Quality of life problems

There are two major concerns about the quality of life criterion for assessing the value of life. The first is that it is a value-laden and judgement-relative alternative. The second problem is that it relies on subjective rather than objective decision-making, so it is difficult to know when we are getting it right.

Quantity of life problems

There is really only one problem with this position and that is that it cannot work in isolation. Length of life is not identical with a good or valuable life, so quality of life questions emerge.

Sanctity of life problems

Judgements on the basis that life is sanctified leave no room for personal judgement about the value of one's own life, let alone the lives of others. It cannot account for the fact that some of us do feel we have reached the point of suffering beyond endurance or that our lives have so diminished in dignity that only death can restore its value. Disturbing though it is, some people will reach this point. The assumption that all life is sanctified would remove the right of the suffering individual to choose how and when it should end:

Different people, of different religious and ethical beliefs, embrace very different convictions about which way of dying confirms and which contradicts the value of their lives. Some fight against death with every weapon their doctors can devise. Others will do nothing to hasten death even if they pray it will come soon. Still others…want to end their lives when they think that living on, in the only way they can, would disfigure rather than enhance the lives they had created. Some people make the latter choice not just to escape pain. Even if it were possible to eliminate all pain for a dying patient – and frequently that is not possible – that would not end or even much alleviate the anguish some would feel at remaining alive, but intubated, helpless, and often sedated near oblivion.[8]

The stakeholders – who ought to decide?

Where individuals are capable of estimating the value of their own lives we encounter problems of whether they are competent enough to do so and of ensuring that depression or fear is not interfering with their evaluation. The subject is further complicated when decisions are made for people who are not competent to judge for themselves the value of their own lives. In either case the question becomes who ought to decide?

External arbiter

An external arbiter is usually believed to be objective and capable of having a clear picture of the person and the context of his or her life. However, the arbiter might not be objective, to the extent that all judgements are based on values and external arbiters will be affected by their own values in making the determination. In addition, given that this person is not the same person whose life is under consideration, he or she might not be able to truly know what is best for the patient. Generally speaking, it feels like a counterintuitive imposition to assume that any one person can make a decision about the value of another person's life.

The main concern is that decisions about the value of another person's life would deteriorate into general assertions about the devaluation of similar lives, as expressed by the concerns in this quote about the value of life of a disabled child:

> I cannot accept [the parent's] view that Stephen would be better off dead. If it is to be decided that 'it is in the best interests of Stephen Dawson that his existence cease', then it must be decided that, for him, non-existence is the better alternative. This would mean regarding the life of a handicapped child as not only less valuable than the life of a normal child, but so much less valuable that it is not worth preserving. I tremble at contemplating the consequences if the lives of disabled persons are dependent upon such judgements.[9]

The example of parenthood reveals that it might be impossible to escape the need for an external arbiter when individuals are not competent to decide for themselves. Neonates, severely disabled or demented persons and people in a persistent vegetative state will not be able to make this choice for themselves.[10] Parents and loved ones are frequently left with the burden of deciding what to do in these tragic situations. In certain cases these decisions clash with established expectations, as they did in the following case.

Case 25
Who decides? Samuel Linares[11]

Five-month-old Samuel Linares aspirated a blue balloon at a birthday party on 2 August, 1988. Paramedics removed the balloon with forceps.

Samuel was left comatose and respirator-dependent in a persistent vegetative state at Chicago's Rush–Presbyterian–St-Luke's Medical Center. When the prognosis became clear, the family asked that the respirator be disconnected and their son allowed to die.

Although the physicians were sympathetic, the hospital's lawyer read federal law to require the hospital to continue treatment to avoid liability for 'murder or child abuse'. The hospital does not have an ethics committee or ethics consultant.

Samuel Linares was going to be moved to a nursing home, despite his family's protests. On 25 April 1988, the night before Samuel was to be moved the distraught father went to the hospital. Mr Linares removed his son from the ventilator, revealing a .357 Magnum when nurses attempted to intervene. Saying, 'I'm not here to hurt anybody', he allowed staff to remove three children from the ICU. His son died in his arms 10 minutes later. Mr Linares confirmed the death with a stethoscope that a doctor slid across the floor. The weeping father surrendered the baby and the gun. Later he said, 'I did it because I love my son and my wife.'

The problem of who decides is made poignantly clear by the seemingly somewhat exaggerated case of the Linares family, but the events described are true. It is not the first time that the best interests of the patient were not obvious, or where agreement could not easily be found.

Consider how a deontologist and a consequentialist would have responded under similar circumstances.

Internal

Permitting individuals to determine the value of their own lives preserves autonomy and reduces the likelihood of coercion. However, it could be too subjective, especially when the person is hindered from making a rational decision by fear and

illness. Nevertheless, it is the best choice because no one can decide for another person what is the best quality of life.

Perhaps the ideal is to let people make their own decisions about the way the quality of their lives affects what quantity they have left. If they perceive their own lives to be sanctified despite any diminishment in quality then that is their own decision. If they prefer to see their lives of such low quality that they seek to reduce or eliminate it altogether, then they ought to be given the assistance they require to ensure that it improves or at least meets the values and hopes they desire. Related reflections are made in Chapter 5 on end of life issues.

Conclusion

We have considered the ideas of quality, quantity and sanctity as they relate to the value of life. These were revealed to have advantages and disadvantages in their application.

Consideration was also given to who ought to determine the value of a given life. External and internal arbiters were considered with the conclusion that it is always safest to permit people to judge for themselves what value to give to their own life.

Notes and references

1 Weber LJ. Who shall live? In: Walter J, Shannon T, eds. Quality of life: the new medical dilemma. New York: Paulist Press; 1990:111–118.
2 Dworkin R et al. Assisted suicide: the philosopher's brief. New York Review of Books; 27 March 1997. Available from On-line Archives: http://www.nybooks.com:6900/nyrev/WWWfeatdisplay.cgi?1997032741F@p1
3 MacIntyre S. Social and psychological issues associated with the new genetics. Phil Trans R Soc London B 1997; 352:1095–1101.
4 See Fish v. Wilcox and Gwent Health Authority; Court of Appeal. [1994] 5 Med LR 230, 13 BMLR 134 as cited in Nelson-Jones R, Burton F. Medical negligence case law. 2nd edn. London: Butterworths; 1995:332–333.

5 Downie R, Calman K. Healthy respect. Oxford: Oxford University Press; 204.

6 Weber LJ. Who shall live? In: Walter J, Shannon T, eds. Quality of life: the new medical dilemma. New York: Paulist Press; 1990:111–118.

7 United Nations High Commissioner For Human Rights: Universal Declaration of Human Rights. Available: http://www.unhchr.ch/udhr/lang/eng.htm

8 Dworkin R et al. Assisted suicide: the philosopher's brief. New York Review of Books; 27 March 1997. Available from On-line Archives: http://www.nybooks.com:6900/nyrev/WWWfeatdisplay.cgi?1997032741F@p1

9 Justice McKenzie BC. Quoted in: Thomas J, Waluchow W. Well and good: case studies in biomedical ethics. Peterborough, Ontario: Broadview Press; 1990.

10 McHaffie HE, Fowlie PW. Life, death and decisions: doctors and nurses reflect on neonatal practice. Hochland & Hochland Ltd; 1996.

11 Miles SH. Hastings Centre Report. July/August 1989:4.

7

Medical audit and medical research

Medical research is fundamental to medical practice. Despite this, medical research often induces an uncomfortable reaction in us when we are patients. This reaction can be attributed to the painful fact, for individuals who might have only just become patients, that the 'perfect' treatment for their condition is not known, and that medical knowledge is incomplete. Despite this, many (in fact, in the experience of the author as a medical researcher, most) patients are prepared to consider participating in medical research, particularly if their participation is explained in terms of their being collaborators in the project. Yet often, when individuals realize that their treatment will be determined randomly, between a conventional and a new therapy or between an active and an inactive agent (placebo), they find this difficult to accept. At the same time, not all patients want to exercise their own choice about their treatment. Especially in life-threatening diseases, some patients prefer their doctor to guide them firmly to the treatment they are to receive.

Ethically and legally, for patients to be recruited to participation in a 'trial' (for example, a randomized controlled trial) researching a novel therapy, equipoise must exist. This means that the medical profession must be as certain as it is possible to be that there is no proof that the novel therapy is more effective than nothing, than placebo or than the accepted standard agent already in use.

The recognition that many time-honoured conventional therapies are inadequate, e.g. are followed by a high proportion of relapses, is a strong motivation to doctors to try to improve things for their patients. To do this necessitates looking for and evaluating novel therapies. These, however, might have downsides that cannot be anticipated. For example, in some, side-effects, in others, adverse drug interactions or very long-term harmful effects that can be identified only if the experimental agent is successful in prolonging life sufficiently for long-term sequelae to occur and be recognized. Interestingly, there is unequivocal evidence that patients with life-limiting disorders who participate in controlled clinical trials do better than similarly affected individuals treated 'off' trials, i.e. outwith any defined treatment protocol.[1] So, whether patients are the type who want their doctor to choose their management, or are the type who want active involvement in the choice of that management, participation in a clinical trial in which genuine equipoise exists can be the 'treatment of choice'. The amount of information given to patients about the trial can be tailored to what they signify to the doctor–researcher is what they want to know.

Medical practice is both empirical and pragmatic. Complete reliance on empirical observation (i.e. relying solely on personal experience) and neglecting previously recorded knowledge is defined as 'quackery'.[2] In practice, because of the idiosyncratic individuality of each person, medical practice is always, to some extent, experimental. This is one reason for careful, consistent recording by doctors of case features, interventions and responses to these by individual patients. This has two advantages. First, it builds up clinical experience, which is of value to the individual practitioner; when shared with others, is of value to colleagues; and, when published, is of value to the profession and society as a whole. Second, it provides the basis for audit, which is the regular comparison of one's own results with those of others managing comparable cases. Audit is not strictly research, although ethical issues that apply to research also apply to audit (e.g., where specified, anonymity of identity of individual participants).[3] Audit is the monitoring of both process and outcome of medical practice, whereas the term 'medical research' carries connotations both of experiment and of innovation, as well as of enlarging medical knowledge and understanding.

There is no doubt that research in medicine is a highly valuable and laudable endeavour, yet certain suspicions persist, founded on well-known concerns about the activities and procedures related to medical research. The intention of this chapter is to examine some of the concerns all researchers have about their practices so as to help potential researchers and research participants better understand the reasons behind existing guidelines and laws governing ethically sound research practice.

A history for concern

Physiological experiments in animals have been part of Western medicine since the eighteenth century. Many of these animal experiments enhanced the understanding by medical practitioners of basic body functions, such as the function of the heart, maintenance of blood pressure, control of circulation and neuromuscular transmission of stimuli. Charles Bell, whose name is commemorated in the condition of facial nerve impairment 'Bell's palsy', wrote in 1815 that, although vivisection enhanced knowledge of bodily function, the inflicting of pain and suffering on animals (which was necessary in that pre-anaesthetic era) was distasteful to him.[4] This repugnance caused him to delay, even permanently postpone, certain animal experiments he felt he needed to do in order

to understand better the function of the human nervous system. In one of his letters he wrote:

> I should be writing a third paper on the Nerves, but I cannot proceed without making some experiments which are so unpleasant to make that I defer them. You may think me silly, but I cannot perfectly convince myself that I am authorised in nature, or religion, to do these cruelties – for what? – for anything else than a little egotism or self-aggrandisement; and yet, what are my experiments in comparison with those that are daily done? And are done for nothing.[4]

Conducting experiments on animals has been paralleled by experimentation on human beings. A literary view of such experimentation comes from Frankenstein's monster, whose very existence was the result of an

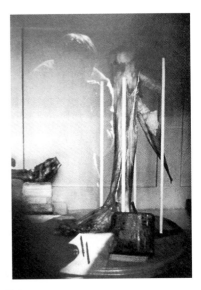

Figure 7.1
Photograph taken with a spy camera while pretending to draw in the Anatomical Museum, Montpelier, France. ('Cet être la, c'est à toi de le créer! Vous devez le créer!' Christine Borland 1997. © Christine Borland. Reprinted with permission of the artist.)

experiment by his scientist creator. As the monster comes to the end of his existence he 'cried with sad and solemn enthusiasm "But soon I shall die, and what I now feel be no longer felt. Soon these burning miseries will be extinct"'.[5]

Evidence of research using human beings exists in the anatomical history museums of colonizing countries. Figure 7.1 is an artistic vision of appropriated specimens of human limbs and torsos, which raises questions about the moral transgressions involved. Figure 7.2 represents the unauthorized appropriation of body cells from Henrietta Laks, who died of cancer in the 1950s.

During the nineteenth and twentieth centuries, humans who were incarcerated as criminals, and those who, as such, were condemned to execution, were quite frequently experimented upon. There are two notable examples from the twentieth century in which humans were treated like, and arguably worse than, animals in medical experiments. One of these examples was the 'research' headed by Dr Josef Mengele on Jews in concentration camps in Germany in the 1940s. An example comes from the novel by Leon Uris entitled *QB VII*. The situations that occur in this book are drawn from real cases, as described by survivors, and offer a true account of 'medical research' on human beings:

> 'I was transferred to Barrack III which held the raw material for the experiments. At first I was to look after six younger Dutch boys who had their testicles irradiated by prolonged exposure to X-ray. It was part of an experiment to sterilise all the Jews...It seems they had X-rayed a number of young women also.'

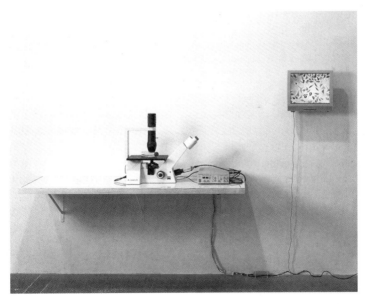

Figure 7.2
This piece illustrates the appropriation of cells from Henrietta Laks, an African–American woman who died of cancer in the 1950s. Her cells were collected exclusively for diagnostic purposes but, because they reproduce so rapidly, they are now used for research worldwide and can be purchased through laboratory catalogues for a small fee. Consent for their use in research was never sought. ('HeLa Hot' Christine Borland 2001 © Christine Borland. Courtesy of the artist and Sean Kelly Gallery, New York.)

'In the evening of November 10th 1943,' Van Damn's voice shook 'fourteen of us were taken from Barrack III to Barrack V. Eight men, six women. I was the first to go. You see, Mr Cady, I am a eunuch. Adam Kelno removed both my testicles....'. 'You were healthy when he did this?' Alexander asked. 'Yes'.[6]

The second example took place in Tuskegee in the American state of Alabama,[7] where approximately 400 men with syphilis had adequate treatment withheld in order to observe and document the natural history of that disease and how it affected African–American sufferers. The aims of the study sounded, and may have been, altruistic and well intended, as explained in the case below.

Case 26
The Tuskegee Syphilis Study

In 1932, the US Public Health Service began working with the then Tuskegee Institute to record the natural history of syphilis. The aim was to try to justify programmes of treatment for African–Americans affected with this disease. The research was entitled the 'Tuskegee Study of Untreated Syphilis in the Negro Male'. The stated aim of the study was to justify a programme of treatment for syphilis in a defined population of individuals who might have been especially at high risk of this disease, and who were too poor to be able to afford healthcare.

Do you think that the motivation for this research was, at face value, beneficent?

The study involved a total of 600 men, of whom approximately 400 were firmly diagnosed as having syphilis, and 200 who did not have evidence of the disease at the outset of the study. The researchers informed all the participants in the study that they were suffering from 'bad blood'. This term was used because it was believed that the participants would not understand the meaning of the term 'syphilis' and so, to make information accessible, the researchers used a term they knew the participants were familiar with, although at the time, in that locality of Alabama, 'bad blood' was in common use for a number of ailments, including (but not just) syphilis.

Do you think that the information given to the participants was appropriate? Is there any problem morally, and practically, with informing all the participating individuals that they had the same diagnosis 'bad blood'?

The fact that syphilis is a venereal disease was perfectly well known when the project was started. The failure of the researchers to inform the participants of the explicit nature of the disease they had would have left those individuals, and their families, unaware of the serious infectious and lethal consequences of being affected by it. The 'controls' also were misinformed because they were grouped with men who had a morbid disease, which at that time was incurable. The controls, as well as their relatives, would have seen infected participants becoming progressively more ill, and might well have worried that, as time went on, they too would become similarly sick and likely to die prematurely. Here is an example where doctors used a euphemism, in a manner that constituted lying, whereby patients, controls and the relatives of both were harmed. In addition, the research subjects could not have given informed consent for their participation in the study, specifically because they were unaware of the true name and nature of the disease under research (see Chapter 3, p. 51).

The subjects did, however, receive something for their participation in the research.

Case 26 continued…
Rewards

Incentives were offered for participating in the study. These were free medical examinations, free meals and complimentary insurance for burial after death. The project was originally planned to last for 6 months; in the event, the Tuskegee Study continued for 40 years.

The offer of incentives or 'rewards' for participating in medical research must always be viewed with caution and scepticism. For the researcher, the morality of needing to persuade participants suggests some coercion. For the participant, if a reward is offered, the question must be asked 'in exchange for what'. In the Tuskegee case, the researchers 'bought' the rights of the participants to receive medical interventions for their conditions. This applied both to those affected by syphilis and to the 'controls'. Although it is accepted that, in the 1930s, before penicillin was discovered and commercially available, syphilis could not be cured, once this antibiotic became available and recognized as a remedy for syphilis, the infected subjects in the Tuskegee Study became morally entitled to treatment with this medication. In the event, it took over 20 years for this to be considered. Clearly, by being participants in this research, these individuals were disadvantaged over a lengthy period of time.

As well as the protracted disadvantages suffered by the participants, further long-term adverse effects for American public health and for African–American society resulted from the unethical research practice at Tuskegee. One of these was the loss of trust in government-initiated public health initiatives (such as might be mounted for AIDS). Another was the development of scepticism towards participation in research, especially among financially and socially deprived individuals who could view themselves as potential victims of ignorant or corrupt research institutions. The potential victims themselves, as well as the community at large, are further victimized because they will miss the benefits that might come from these initiatives.

Guidance and solutions

The fact that Mengele's experiments and the Tuskegee study were done in the name of medical research[8] makes it desirable, even essential, that healthcare professionals think systematically about the ethical issues relevant to medical research. Encouraging patient involvement in medical research can help this. 'Action research', where individuals affected by particular disorders approach healthcare providers and researchers who are studying their condition, is a phenomenon where the patients' interests are likely to be held in the forefront. The recent trend for 'consumer involvement' in the steering groups for medical research projects is a further important factor that should influence favourably the deserts, needs and rights of the participants, particularly when these are patients.[9]

What basic ethical principles can you think of which have a bearing on ensuring that medical research is ethical?

Basic ethical principles described in Chapter 1 (p. 8) provide a starting point for the consideration of the ethics of medical research. The four principles of Beauchamp and Childress[10] are useful foundations here: autonomy, beneficence, non-maleficence and justice. Simple application of any one of these to the two examples of the medical experiments cited above demonstrates that they are unethical. Application of the four principles together shows that those experiments were unethical on all counts. However, a dubious utilitarian justification can be made by claiming that the greater good was achieved because the public health of society at large was enhanced, even though it was at the harsh expense of the relatively smaller numbers of people; namely the Jewish subjects experimented on by Mengele, and the 600 African–American subjects in the Tuskegee Syphilis Study. This demonstrates the observation that a paraphrase for utilitarianism is 'the end justifies the means'; a corollary that is strongly criticized for the immoral outcomes it can be used to justify. It is also a stark illustration of the potential dangers of unthinking application of the utilitarian theory to medical ethics. This frequently utilized tool in the armament of administrators, managers and politicians often appeals to the public, as clients, consumers and voters.

In contrast, deontological perspectives would strongly condemn the utilitarian justification (in the spirit of Pappworth[11] quoted in Chapter 3, p. 61). A deontological perspective would state that a duty of care is owed by researchers to participants, and that respect for individual liberty *must* precede community benefits. Without this duty-based safeguard there is nothing to prevent the exploitation of human beings in the context of research.

It was in the aftermath of the Holocaust (1933–1945) and the Second World War that legislation to regulate medical research gained significant momentum. It is considered that the first international code of ethics governing human experimentation is the Nuremberg Code of 1947,[12] which defined ten elements that should be observed in medical research on humans (see Appendix 4).

What principles would you observe if you were going to carry out research on humans?

Ironically, Nuremberg was the place and the name given to the first formulation by the German Nazi regime of its anti-Semitic laws, which were drawn up in 1935. The Nuremberg Code was part of the judgement summing up the Nazi war crimes Trials that were held in Nuremberg after the Second World War.[13] The ethical principles governing medical research were formally adopted by the medical profession under the auspices of the World Medical Association in 1964 in a document called the Declaration of Helsinki (see Appendix 6). This document has been reviewed regularly, such that revised versions have appeared from time to time. The version current at the time of publication of this book was approved by the World Medical Association and published in 2000. Subsequently, a number of codes, declarations and guidelines have been published, including by the Medical Research Councils of Britain[14] and of Canada, the NHS, the Royal College of Nurses, the Council of the Professions Allied to Medicine, the Royal College of Physicians, the United States Food and Drug Administration, the United Nations, the International Conference on Harmonisation, and a number from meetings of the World Medical Association in different venues at different times, e.g. Tokyo 1975 and Lisbon 1996.

More recently, the Nuffield Council for Bioethics, which is based in London, has begun to consider guidelines for ethical research for projects from affluent countries that involve testing interventions on participants from post-colonial nations facing great economic hardship. This opens broader questions about power relationships between countries that go beyond the scope of this chapter, although some are addressed in Chapter 9.

Historically, there have been arguments and controversies generated within the medical profession by calls for defined ethical standards. Indeed, it was not until 1978 that the General Medical Council was required by law to issue such standards.[15] Leaders of the profession and of professional organizations have been reluctant to initiate and foster guidelines and recommendations on ethical practice in medical research.[16] Usually this is not because of a desire to hide unethical behaviour but because of concern that too many restrictions would inhibit and even prevent useful research from being done. This is why many codes of ethics are broad and not enforced as laws but only as guidelines that can be questioned. As a result, the codes are perhaps not wholly adequate for providing absolute answers to moral confusions of researchers who only want to do the right thing. However, they do provide guidance and act as points of reference for debates on best practice. They can also be breached, but the onus is on researchers who reject an ethical code to justify their choice of action. Currently much more widely seen as appropriate for students and trainee doctors, some of the many codes and declarations that have been issued need to be interpreted for the here and now to make them relevant to the particular experiment or research project proposed at the moment. To analyse for practical use the ethics of medical research, it is useful to define categories and then to discuss 'special cases', particularly vulnerable client groups such as children, those who are physically or psychologically incapacitated and adults who are 'incompetent' (see Chapter 2, p. 25).

Types of medical research

Uncontrolled and controlled trials

> How many different types of medical research can you think of?

The range of different types of medical research is wide. As alluded to at the beginning of this chapter, at the basic level of the one-to-one doctor–patient relationship, any intervention – pharmacological, physical or psychological – can be and is experimental, albeit not regularly classified as research. Where the intervention is new, i.e. previously unevaluated, there is an element of research

about it. Should the patient be informed of this? Should the patient be given the opportunity to decline to receive innovative or untried treatments? The codes of research ethics are clear in their answers to both these questions: Yes!

From the 'one doctor with one patient' interaction, we move on to therapy for groups of individuals. Such interventions are called trials. Classically, four levels of these are recognized.

Uncontrolled trials
Uncontrolled trials monitor the progress of a disease in a single group of patients only. In other words, there is no comparison or control group of subjects. The ethical justification for such studies is that the information gleaned from them is highly relevant to a limited group. For example, the ability to tolerate the new agent by individuals with the condition for which it had been designed could be determined. Only after such a general level of toleration has been observed is it ethical to proceed to comparisons of the new agent with any already-accepted therapies. Such uncontrolled trials can be conducted on relatively small numbers of affected individuals, which is in itself an ethical justification for running them, because only small numbers of individuals are put at risk. On utilitarian grounds, it is ethically preferable to expose smaller numbers of patients to uncertain effects before launching into larger comparative studies, which, to achieve statistical significance, require larger numbers of subjects.

Controlled trials
Four levels of controlled trial are recognized, often called Phase 1, Phase 2, Phase 3 and Phase 4 trials (see Appendix 5). Strict codes and protocols exist for inviting and recruiting patients to all of these.

> In what ways might a doctor inadvertently coerce a potential patient to participate in a treatment trial?

In all cases, the ethical principles that guide clinical trials ensure that the patients:

- know their treatment is being delivered in the context of a trial
- are informed, as far as is foreseeable, of possible side-effects
- participate voluntarily (i.e. without coercion)
- are free to withdraw from the treatment at any time
- need *not* give a reason for withdrawing
- maintain their former relationship with their doctors; i.e. the trial does not prejudice this relationship.

Although individuals allocated to the control group appear at first glance to be disadvantaged, in fact more extended consideration indicates that they are being managed as justly as the individuals randomized to the active therapy; e.g. they will be spared unforeseen dangerous or toxic side-effects. So, in a situation where the trial turns out to have a negative result, the patients who received placebo have been spared any adverse effects, which those in the intervention arm were necessarily exposed to. At the end of the trial, that suffering could even reveal itself to be to no avail, if the treatment proves ineffective. It is worth emphasizing that it is only morally right to use a placebo, or a 'no treatment arm', in a clinical trial where, for all practical purposes, there is very strong evidence that absolutely no efficacious treatment is in existence. In the Tuskegee Study (see p. 124), while there was no curative treatment available for syphilis, from 1932 to 1947, there was some justification for an observational study of no treatment. However, once penicillin was available, and even while it was thought to be *potentially* curative, the equipoise of the study was lost and it became unethical to continue without offering treatment. This example illustrates the necessity for regular review of ongoing clinical trials, although even this can lead to problems because premature breaking of codes in such studies can result in a whole extensive project becoming valueless. However, the Tuskegee example illustrates that regular review of the context, and of parallel developments, would

have been beneficial to the participants and to the triallists. Much less harm would have been done, and more good achieved, with greater justice resulting all round.

Therapeutic and non-therapeutic trials
Clinical trials make up a substantial proportion of formal medical research that sets out to evaluate the efficacy of therapy. As the therapeutic interventions have the purpose of modulating disease processes and the signs and symptoms caused by these, administration of the interventions is appropriate only to individuals manifesting these conditions and disorders.

In the process of seeking knowledge about human physiology, medical research can be, and is, done on healthy volunteers. This is non-therapeutic research, and is a pragmatic endeavour. Strong deontological considerations prevail, with duty of care at the centre of this utilitarian activity. These healthy participants are entitled to consideration by the researcher in regard to all of the fundamental 'big four' ethical principles: autonomy, beneficence, non-maleficence and justice (see Chapter 1, p. 8).

The voluntary aspect of participation demonstrates the **autonomy**. With volunteers who are healthy, the **beneficence** towards the participants is less evident because the exercise does not set out to 'improve' their health or their quality of life. In contrast, the **non-maleficence** component is very prominent because it is mandatory that medical research on healthy volunteers does them no harm or, if any harm is done, it is reversible and anticipated and so prepared for by both parties involved. An example would be where a volunteer has no history of allergy and is to receive a medication that, on the basis of its chemistry, is unlikely to be allergenic. The volunteer would need to be aware that exposure of humans to any new substance can, in theory, induce an allergic response. The researcher would need to be prepared for this unlikely possibility by having adequate trained staff, as well as drugs like antihistamines, adrenaline and corticosteroids at hand, so that the volunteer could be rescued from a potentially disastrous complication such as anaphylactic shock. Ensuring **justice** embraces consideration of the first three principles but extends to recognition of services and time given by the volunteer to the research project, as well as the researcher providing reasonable remuneration for costs of travel and other expenses necessarily incurred. For all these reasons, non-therapeutic trials are usually only performed on competent adults who by definition are able to give their consent to their participation. Non-therapeutic interventions should not involve incapacitated people who are unable to consider the risks (such as exemplified above), and unable to weigh whether they are willing to undertake these. For incapacitated people to participate in trials, it must be demonstrated that this participation is potentially to the advantage of people with their type of incapacity. Clearly, this cannot be the case in non-therapeutic studies.

Non-interventionist research

Case 27
The research questionnaire

Dear Dr Neil,
I recently received a request from you to fill in a questionnaire regarding the treatment I underwent for breast cancer last year. Since I regard information related to my health to be private, I would like to know how you discovered that I have breast cancer and how you came to have access to this information, including my name and address.

I am generally in favour of medical research and usually consider it my duty to participate. However, I believe it is common practice to receive permission from research subjects before hand, and I do not recall giving my consent to having my personal records examined by you.

Yours in good faith
Mrs B. Thomson

As well as the three types of therapeutic research discussed above, namely individual, cohort, and healthy volunteer studies, other types of medical research are undertaken studying case notes and disease registries. These forms of medical research generate data that contribute enormously to the knowledge and understanding of human disease. Indeed, the disciplines of epidemiology and of public health almost owe their existence to the capacity to pursue knowledge in this way. Comprehension of disease processes and patient management in all disciplines is informed and sustained by such information. Despite its importance, the collection of such information must respect the autonomy and privacy of the individuals whose conditions and status constitute the statistics that provide the overview. The ideal for collecting epidemiological data is that individuals agree that their biographical and biological information will be collected and incorporated into research reports. For these activities, individuals can be reassured that their identity will be rendered anonymous and that the data accumulated is used only for good and moral purposes. This means the data will be used for the greater good of society and not solely for the profit or advancement of the data gatherer or registrar. In the UK, the Data Protection Act (1998) encoded these requirements as rights for individuals for data stored electronically; this will soon be extended to ensure these rights for manually stored data. In practice, the obtaining of permission for registering many medical conditions that are rated by the community as worth recording does not always happen. Here, weighing of merits has to occur. Society as a whole has to decide whether the benefits weigh more heavily than the disadvantages of not registering data for which formal permission has not been obtained. This is an ongoing debate.

What do you think? Do the benefits of cancer registries outweigh the fact that individuals on these have not given their explicit permission?

Can these arguments extend to other conditions as well? (See p. 34 and 42.)

An example of the information that cancer registries produce is the death rates from cancer of particular organs between different geographical areas, or between workers in different occupations.

Where medical research is done by accessing patient case records, the confidentiality and security of these must be guaranteed; i.e. the researcher must ensure that, when work is published, no individuals whose records have been studied can be identified. A practical consideration to ensure the welfare of patients on those occasions when their records are being studied in a research programme, is to make sure that the case notes can be obtained quickly should the clinical needs of the patient require them for treatment. Their exact whereabouts should be indicated on a tracer card in the Medical Records department stack. Such case notes must be accessible by the staff of the Medical Records department at any time of day or night.

Medical research in those who are especially vulnerable

In an earlier chapter, we considered the fact that special considerations exist in the clinical relationships of doctors with three groups of especially vulnerable individuals: (i) minors; (ii) those with mental disabilities; and (iii) those with diminished capabilities, e.g. those who are temporarily or permanently 'incompetent'. A fourth group is those who are dying. These four groups of especially vulnerable individuals also require special consideration when medical research with them is being proposed.

Medical research in minors

Two basic facts make research in minors desirable, even essential. First, many of the disorders and diseases that manifest in children are unique to their distinctive stages of development. For example, haemolytic jaundice in newborn babies is a condition unique to neonates. Second, the biological, biochemical and physiological phenomena associated with health and life in minors are different from the same phenomena in adults. This is illustrated by the fact that the normal respiratory rate per minute in a 1-year-old child is 30 breaths per minute, compared with 12 breaths per minute in a healthy resting adult. To determine the effectiveness of medical interventions for disorders in these subjects, the evaluations can be meaningfully pursued only in affected minors.

In the chapter on consent, it emerged that the validity of consent from a minor for a medical intervention depended upon the physician being satisfied that the individual child concerned had sufficient maturity and understanding to be able to appreciate the nature and consequences of the intervention. In the UK, investing jurisdiction concerning 'Gillick competence' on the medical practitioner actually involved with the minor (see Chapter 2, p. 26), both imbues the doctor with considerable influence and simultaneously requires the doctor to practise considerable prudence (i.e. knowledge, scholarship and wisdom). In therapy, these onerous responsibilities concerning competence in children (minors) are vested by society and the courts chiefly on the doctor responsible for the intervention. This is also the situation when seeking consent for participation in medical research by minors in the UK. It is clear, however, that in the research context the responsible physician could be less detached because of a vested interest in pursuing the research. This could make the researcher less arbitrary in making the judgement as to whether a minor has the maturity and understanding to consent to participate in the research. Natural justice, as well as regulation, requires that checks and balances are in place to regulate the recruitment of minors into medical research.

Guidelines for research in minors are usually available from the organizations that regulate the involvement of adults in medical research. These include the General Medical Council, the Medical Research Councils of Britain and of Canada, the Royal College of Physicians and the World Medical Association.

In his handbook of good practice entitled *Ethics in Medial Research*,[17] Trevor Smith, writing about medical research in vulnerable groups, states that clinicians should think and talk about medical research *with* rather than *in* children. This simple change in preposition reveals a vast shift in attitude on the part of the researcher. 'With' indicates collaboration, common good, respect and sensitivity – valuable ideals that are applicable in any research context. These attitudes are extensions of other good attitudes that Smith advocates for the medical researcher inviting patients to participate in this. He suggests that conscience and intuition should come into play to create fairness, openness and altruism in this activity. The core governing duty in research involving children is that the intervention must be in the best interest of the child. For this reason, non-therapeutic research involving children cannot be done because it does not benefit the child directly. The best interests of the individual child *must* prevail.

Medical research in those with mental disabilities

Just as medical research of paediatric conditions can usually be pursued only in children, so medical research of neurological and psychiatric conditions can often be pursued only in patients with these conditions. In common debilitating mental disorders, such as depression or schizophrenia, individuals affected by these conditions are vulnerable. Despite this, Trevor Smith argues that such subjects should be included in research into these disabilities, because they stand uniquely to benefit from positive

results of such research. Whether it is ethical for such people to be included in research that is not directly relevant to their psychiatric condition seems questionable, although if they express a wish so to do, and the doctor considers they have the capacity to consent, their inclusion could be legitimate. This would seem to be an area of special sensitivity, where determination of capacity might more fairly and safely be undertaken by more than one professional, preferably independent of the research.[18]

Society sees few problems with medical research into common physical morbidity-inducing conditions like cancer and coronary artery disease. Indeed, such research attracts huge popular support. Surely, in principle, there is no difference in the case for research into mental disorders, except the difficulty of obtaining free and valid consent. All the features described above for seeking consent to participate in research from non-vulnerable subjects apply, except that occasionally in mental illness the nature of the studies require that some facts about these will be intentionally withheld from participants until studies are finished. Consciousness of the need for quality communication and for respect for others (both patients and fellow professionals) is underlined in another 'good practice' point by Trevor Smith, writing about research with psychiatric patients. He recommends that in studies in which questionnaire-type inventories are used to indicate possible emotional/psychological pathology, pre-study consent for their use should emphasize for the participant that where these instruments reveal possible pathology, both the patient and the patient's medical adviser will be informed of the finding.

Medical research in incompetent adults

Several of the principles arising about research in minors and the mentally disabled or incapacitated also apply to adults with physical incapacity. A frequently encountered example of where such research is appropriate, where the affected patients stand uniquely to benefit and yet where they can rarely consent, is stroke and other disorders that result in sudden collapse and complete or near complete mental and physical incapacity. One feature of medical research with these situations is the pressing requirement implicit in the nature of their conditions that medical interventions occur as quickly as possible, because the patients are in urgent need. The catastrophic nature of these conditions for individuals affected by them, and for their relatives, makes it vital that these conditions should not be precluded from that medical research by which, uniquely, they can be better understood and managed.

At present there are few, if any, administrative or legal protocols in the UK to guide researchers or protect patients. Both the parties are provided for by the requirement that all clinical research is submitted to and passed by Local Research Ethics Committees (LRECS) and, for nationwide studies, Multicentre Research Ethics Committees (MRECS). This requirement does not pertain exclusively to incapacitated participants. Ethics committees are discussed in more detail later in this chapter (see p. 134). The other contemporary initiative relevant to these conditions is the public debate, and indeed advocacy by some groups, of advance directives ('living wills' described in Chapter 5, p. 97).

Although both consent by an ethics committee and the provisions of an advance directive can assist in the decision as to whether an acutely incapacitated adult should be managed in a research setting (e.g. a clinical trial), the decision might in practice have to be made by the responsible medical practitioner or even the medical practitioner of first contact, e.g. a casualty officer or a house officer. Normal etiquette, as well as good practice, indicate that, where they exist and can be contacted, relatives' views should be sought. However, the doctor involved has

to bear in mind that the relatives might not be sufficiently knowledgeable about the patient nor, in the circumstances, emotionally equipped to make a decision. At present, under British law, the views of the relatives about these matters carry little weight (in Scotland, legislative work is currently being pursued to address some of these uncertainties in the Adults with Incapacities [Scotland] Act 2000).[18] One further consideration about consent from a relative for participation in research by a related patient is that, in the circumstances of an adverse outcome, the relative who was consulted and acquiesced to participation in the research might feel responsible for, and even guilty about, the outcome. In the nature of such conditions, and in the context of soundly planned, ethically approved studies, a bad outcome cannot possibly be something for which a relative should feel responsible. Responsibility-taking by the doctor reduces the likelihood of inappropriate guilt in relatives.

Some medical conditions of adults that need urgent research are characterized by fluctuating capacity; Alzheimer's disease is a notable example. In these conditions, the valid consent of the patients can frequently be obtained. For such conditions, Smith advises obtaining formally the consent of the relatives as well as of the patients. He says that, despite the irrelevance of this consent in law, it is essential from the ethical viewpoint. It certainly signifies a caring, concerned approach, which evidences willingness on the part of the researcher to communicate with others who have a stake in the conditions of the individuals being treated.

> How can you reconcile issues of breach of confidentiality in seeking 'parallel supporting' consent from relatives of adult patients who have medical conditions characterized by fluctuating capacity (in law 'competence')?

Medical research in the dying

Patients who are reaching the end of their lives often gain a sense of satisfaction from participating in research. They recognize that knowledge discovered on themselves might, in the future, benefit others. When inviting dying patients to participate in such research, where the researcher knows that the impending death is inevitable, it is important when exercising beneficence and non-maleficence that these are not misinterpreted by the patient as indicating that there is hope of prolonging life. In other words, an invitation to dying patients to participate in medical research needs to be couched in terms that in no way raise false hope. Some practitioners feel an awkwardness in seeking consent for participation in research of people who will not benefit from this, particularly where participation could result in inconvenience or added discomfort. These feelings can, and frequently are, balanced by feelings of altruism in the participant. The very fact that individuals being approached have had their right recognized to choose to participate in an activity in which they might help future generations, or members of their own family who might contract the same disease, can be a positive, even heart-warming experience.

Issues to consider

Overall, a healthcare professional who is planning research has a catalogue of issues to address before starting. These include:

- The responsibility not to repeat previously performed research unnecessarily. Circumstances such as differing geographical or different socioeconomic environments justify repetition of some research. Even when these circumstances exist, meticulous, comprehensive searching of literature from all over the world should be done before research is commenced

- The purpose, i.e. what will the research reveal?
- To try to establish that the results will not be trivial
- To ensure that the research is not impractical to achieve
- The motivation; i.e. why do I want to do this research. Is it to enhance my professional standing or to make life better for patients? (If it does the latter, career and reputation of the researcher are likely to be enhanced as well, which is an acceptable spin-off)
- The harmful effects, i.e. who or what might be damaged by my proposed research? Not all adverse effects of innovative management can be determined in advance of this being tried out for real. Indeed, a purpose of much medical research is to establish if such effects will occur, and whether they outweigh the benefits. Nevertheless, there is an onus on the researcher to anticipate any harm the research might cause as imaginatively and as honestly as possible
- Rightful ownership of specimens, i.e. has the person from whom a particular specimen to be used in a research project given permission for that material to be used in this way, including storage for future as yet undefined research?
- Permission, i.e. have my proposals, including those for use and storage of body tissue specimens, been submitted to a research ethics committee, and approved?

Overall for medical research, whether this is individual or cohorts of patients or healthy volunteers, whether this is therapeutic or observational, respect for the personhood of individuals being researched is basic. From this will flow recognition of their autonomy; their freedom to participate or not; their entitlement to clearly worded, honest accounts of what their participation in the research will involve, and of possible adverse effects to anticipate. When considering these, the researchers need to exercise their imaginations. A good way of doing this is for them to put themselves into their patients' shoes, as Sir Hedley Atkins did when he initiated trials of treatment of operable breast cancer in the 1930s at Guy's Hospital in London. Before a trial was launched, all members of the multi-disciplinary team had to signify that they personally would be agreeable to themselves or their next of kin participating in the study.

Chapter 3 (p. 42) mentioned the fact that, in the context of medical research, the participants need to be aware that they can withdraw at any time, without fear of rebuke from their carers or their peers. Researchers need to recognize that continual consent is necessary for continuous participation in a research programme or trial.

Research Ethics Committees

Research Ethics Committees provide multidisciplinary peer review of research proposals. They create a consistent structure into which such proposals have to be presented. This serves to ensure comprehensiveness in preparation of research proposals.[19] It also brings these into the public view, which is intended to prevent dubious, inadequate and, even more importantly, immoral and unsound research proceeding. Participants as well as practitioners are protected by the existence of Research Ethics Committees. Research that has not been approved by a Research Ethics Committee (even if such yields 'good' findings) is most unlikely to be accepted for publication in a reputable scholarly journal. This is in compliance with a steadily widening international agreement between publishers of medical and scientific journals. The existence of abuses and abominations in medical research described earlier in this chapter point to the rightness of this practice, even though it could result in some good research not being either undertaken or publicized.

There are two types of research ethics committees in the UK, local and multicentre.

There are two subtypes of local research ethics committee. One of these is based in a hospital and the other in the community, for community and primary care research. Their responsibility is to review submitted research proposals that will take place in their local area or individual hospitals. The multicentre committees were set up to review proposals for medical research scheduled to occur across a wide geographic area, i.e. involving patients who are recruited from or in several hospitals in different healthcare administrations. Both Local and Multicentre Research Ethics Committees are made up of individuals from differing disciplines. These often include a scientist, or/and a statistician, sometimes a lawyer, a philosopher or a theologian, and always medical and nursing practitioners and lay people. The committees act as a form of peer review for researchers and can help improve or polish proposals and projects.

Conclusions

- Medical research is essential
- Research requires regulation
- Absence of regulation results in abuses
- Rules do not guarantee morality
- The Declaration of Helsinki[20] encodes principles that should govern medical research with humans (see Appendix 6)
- Many organizations have created codes to govern medical research
- Autonomy of the individual is the dominant principle in research
- Patient consent, following full information, is the ideal
- Special vigilance for their welfare is necessary for patients unable to receive information and give consent
- Medical Research Ethics Committees exist in the UK to regulate research. All research involving patients should be approved by such a committee before starting.

Notes and references

1 Gelber RD, Goldhirsch A. Can a clinical trial be the treatment of choice for patients with cancer? J Natl Cancer Inst 1988; 80:886–887.

2 Boyd KM et al. eds. The new dictionary of medical ethics. London: British Medical Journal Publishing Group; 1997.

3 Rogers WA, Braunack-Mayer A. Handling information: some ethical issues. Australian Family Physician 2000; 29(8):806–808.

4 Gordon-Taylor G, Walls EW. Sir Charles Bell, his life and times. Edinburgh: E & S Livingstone; 1958:111.

5 Shelley M. Frankenstein. 1818. Republished 1921 by Everymans Library, London.

6 Uris L. QB VII [Queen's Bench VII] London: Harper Collins; 1992.

7 Jones J. Bad blood: the Tuskegee syphilis experiment. A tragedy of race and medicine. New York: The Free Press; 1981.

8 Centre for Disease Control and Prevention website. Available: http://www.cdc.gov/nchstp/od/tuskegee/time.htm #top

9 Hornblum AM. Acres of skin. New York: Routledge; 1998.

10 Beauchamp TL, Childress JF. The principles of biomedical ethics. 4th edn. Oxford: Oxford University Press; 1994.

11 Pappworth MH. Human guinea pigs. Boston, MA: Beacon Press; 1967.

12 Shuster E. The Nuremberg code: Hippocratic ethics and human rights. Lancet 1998; 351:974–977.

13 Levine RJ. Ethics and regulation of clinical research: Appendix 3. Baltimore, MD: Urban and Schwarzenburg; 1981.

14 Medical Research Council guidelines for good clinical practice in clinical trials. London: MRC Publications; 1998. Available: http://www.mrc.ac.uk/ethics

15 Commonwealth Medical Association. Medical ethics and human rights: report of the CMA project on the role of medical ethics in the protection of human rights: Part 1. London: BMA Publications; 1993–4.

16 Pappworth MH. Human guinea pigs – a history. Br Med J 1990; 301:1456–1460.

17 Smith T. Ethics in medical research: a handbook of good practice. Cambridge: Cambridge University Press; 1999.

18 Adults with Incapacity [Scotland] Act 2000. Available at: http://www.scotland-legislation.hmso.gov.uk/legislation/scotland/acts2000/20000004

19 MREC guidelines for researchers – patient information sheet and consent form. Available: http://dialspace.dial.pipex.com/mrec.pis.htm

20 Helsinki Declaration 2000. Available from the World Medical Association website: www.wma.net

8

Human reproduction and new reproductive technologies

The world of human reproduction has grown increasingly complicated (Fig. 8.1). It was never simple, but attempts to resolve some of its original complications have only made things more complicated. People who don't want to have children now have safe options available to them to prevent and terminate unwanted pregnancies, which raises debates about the correctness of such actions and the rights of those involved. People who want children but cannot produce them naturally now have options of surrogacy and new technologies that lead to accusations of the commodification of children and women and the basic materials it takes to create living human beings. Are these reduced to mere consumer goods, or are we really helping to relieve the suffering of those who cannot or prefer not to have children?

In this chapter we will consider a number of issues related to the debates on several subjects. Because most of the technologies are new there will be fewer answers than questions. Wherever possible, case studies will be used to illustrate the issues under consideration.

Abortion

This was one of the earliest questions to be debated in the field of medical ethics. To

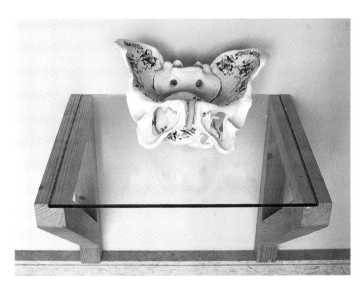

Figure 8.1
The fragility of the china pelvis and infant skull reflects the dangers inherent in childbirth. The title of the sculpture – '5 set conversation pieces' – questions the appropriateness of such sensitive and dangerous matters being discussed casually. ('5 set conversation pieces' Christine Borland 1998 [detail] © Christine Borland. Courtesy of the artist and Sean Kelly Gallery, New York.)

date, there are no resolutions to the debate except possibly a recognition that the various stakeholders will agree to disagree on the ultimate rights or wrongs of abortion. We will try to give fair consideration to a variety of issues raised by this emotive debate. This section will convey some suggested perspectives of the debate as they are manifest in the ethics literature. Abortion is a highly sensitive topic so readers are reminded, even urged, to be especially open-minded and respectful of others' opinions. Doing so will make it easier to reflect on the strengths and weaknesses of the different perspectives in order to formulate justifications to support your own position.

Case 28
Abortion

Mrs K was a 37-year-old woman with four children. Her doctor informed her that she was pregnant after she consulted for irregular periods. Mrs K became very disturbed as soon as her period was overdue. She claimed she already had as many children as she could handle both emotionally and financially. She had always thought abortion was wrong, but now she felt desperate because she did not want another child.

Mrs K was using a diaphragm as contraception, having stopped birth control pills for fear of their ill effects. She had spoken with her husband about abortion and he told her he would support her decision.

The patient saw her physician to ask for a referral for an abortion. She admitted to having thoughts of suicide and self-harm but did not believe she would go through with it. She was also concerned that no one should find out about the pregnancy because she suspected her friends and family would not approve of her choice. She was subsequently referred for an abortion.

In some ways this is a classic case of request for abortion. Women seek abortions for numerous reasons, some of which are considered more acceptable than others. The reasons for accepting or rejecting abortion are complex but many arguments revolve on the premise that the fetus has a right to life. Could it be argued that the fetus Mrs K was carrying had a right to live?

Fetal rights: do they exist?

The simple answer to this question is no. The laws in most countries do not recognize the rights of the fetus. In legal terms, only after an infant is born viable can it be said to hold a right, at which time it is possible for the infant to act as pursuant in a legal case regarding harm or injury in the womb.[1] Note that this is a legal decision and might clash with some people's moral beliefs that the fetus ought to have rights that can be protected.

If we were to grant rights to a fetus then we would need to consider if those rights could supersede the rights of the mother (or anyone else for that matter). The argument seems to be fuelled by two opposing sides. The so-called pro-life supporters tend to claim that the fetus has rights and, because of its helplessness and innocence, these rights have to be protected from any infringement whatsoever. The counterclaim, made by the so-called pro-choice movement, is that absolute observance of fetal rights places the fetus in a superior position to anyone else, because no one has such complete protection of his or her rights. One most obvious example of the limitations of rights is that no one has a right to liberty that includes theft of another person's property. If one person steals from another, the first person's right of freedom is restricted by arrest and imprisonment. Most rights have been compromised in certain contexts, and even rights to life have been overridden when competing rights intervene.

Some people doubt whether the fetus can have rights at all because they do not recognize the fetus as a *person* but rather as a human being or organism. They claim that all fetuses are only *potential* persons but, because they are not rational and have no memories of their own narrative existences, they cannot claim the same status as human beings who *are* persons. On this argument, a fetus can no more bear a right than an acorn can have branches.[2] However, equally problematic are questions of what makes a person or when can a human be identified as possessing what we will call *personhood*? The memory-based criterion outlined above would exclude newborns and comatose or severely demented adults.[3] These human beings would therefore have no rights, or only restricted rights such as those afforded to animals. On the positive side, defining persons as separate from humans does protect other possible non-human persons, such as aliens from another planet or dolphins. This might sound absurd, but it is relevant because otherwise we are assuming that only humans can be persons, which is an inductive argument based solely on never having encountered evidence of other beings besides humans to whom we wish to ascribe the rights and dignities of a person. For all we know, we will someday encounter a being which in no way resembles a human being but which thinks, feels, communicates and remembers in similar ways.

The philosophical concept of personhood

Part of the debate about the rights status of the fetus depends on whether the fetus is considered to be a person as opposed to just a human being. The criteria for personhood are set out in order to protect the possibility that non-human persons can be protected and respected. This is a non-speciesist position and is outlined in the following paragraphs.

Usually, we use the thought experiment of an alien from outer space who is not human in any way but who displays the characteristics of a person. We would want to have respect for this person and have mechanisms for protecting the person's

rights. But why? What criteria would we use to define personhood?

The criteria for personhood are not fixed. Some people draw the line at certain stages of physical development, particularly linked to the development of the central nervous system. Other arguments bar mere physical criteria in favour of less obvious, but more specific conditions. These are not clearly defined but usually include:

- the ability to be rational
- sentience accompanied by intelligence
- memory of an ongoing or continuous self (self-awareness)
- the capacity to be informed
- the capacity of understanding
- the ability to assert judgements and choices.

However, as we have seen, these criteria will necessarily exclude some human beings, including fetuses, newborns, some children, intellectually impaired humans, adults suffering from dementia and comatose humans. So these criteria will not help to establish rights for the fetus, they simply raise more problems.

Ascribing rights to fetuses as *potential* persons is no less problematic because it implies an infinite regression to the absurd conclusion that all human genetic material with the potential to become a person deserves the respect of a person; this would include all unfertilized eggs and sperm. The conclusion is nonsensical because it would require the fertilization of all ova to protect the right of the potential people they could become.

The mother's rights: are they prime?

The language surrounding abortion often refers to the mother's right to choose. Does Mrs K have a right to have an abortion? On the basis of the criteria listed above, mothers can be said to be persons because they have the ability to act rationally and have a developed sense of themselves as continuously existing entities (narrative memory). They are also able to hold their rights in a responsible way and respond to the duties these rights confer in a reciprocal respect of the rights of others. Therefore, there is no doubt that mothers can have rights. The right of the mother most clearly exercised in abortion decisions is her right to bodily integrity. This is a well-recognized right that most people regard as fundamental. The right is supported by laws against assault, which even go as far as to protect people who would refuse to give blood to save another person's life or to help in a murder investigation.

> Should the mother's right to control over her own body be allowed to supersede the possible or potential rights of the fetus?

Pro-life supporters say no, no one has a right that can supersede the right to be born and to live.

Pro-choice supporters say yes, no one can force anyone else to assume the risks and violation of the body involved in a pregnancy (see Bodily integrity, p. 141).[4]

Most importantly, it must be recognized that choosing a termination is one of the most difficult decisions any woman will ever have to make and subsequently live with. The case of Mrs K illustrates how women will choose abortion out of necessity rather than capriciousness or irresponsibility. Most women take the choice of abortion very seriously and do not assume the burden lightly. The image of the 'evil female' who callously disposes of her offspring does not reflect the reality of most women who choose to have an abortion. Some theorists will argue that this image is more likely to be the product of an anxiety about female autonomy, of women having too much control over the process of procreation.[5] Rather than identifying abortion as a right, then, this perspective illuminates an aspect of abortion that shows it as a

burden and enormous responsibility for the women who might need to choose it as an option. Abortion is more legitimately seen as a tragic choice for those who, like Mrs K, feel they have no better alternative. Instead, we ought to consider as a society why it is that women find themselves in a position where they must terminate a pregnancy in order to protect any number of other interests, including the lives of actual children in the woman's care, her career or her social standing. Is it fair for women to have to bear the burden alone?

The father's rights: are they relevant?

One consideration is that the male partner might share this burden of responsibility, but this leads to further complications. Should the father have rights in the case of abortion or are his rights only potential rights, just as he is only a potential father? Such issues are raised primarily when the biological father attempts to block the woman's choice to have an abortion. In the case under consideration, Mr K claims to be supportive of Mrs K's decision. Many people take this position; namely that it is the woman's body and therefore her partner will stand by any choice she makes. This could be out of recognition of her right to bodily integrity or it might be a desire to abdicate responsibility for the outcome.

Now consider, as has been the case in several real life situations,[6] if Mr K was not prepared to accept his wife's choice to have an abortion and attempted to block her from doing so. The rights of mothers and fathers are mutually exclusive when the father does not want the termination but the mother does. If his rights supersede the mother's rights then he is given privilege in the context. Is this appropriate, considering it is she who will have to take all of the bodily risks including violation of her bodily integrity? In the UK the law does not recognize the right of the father to accept or reject an abortion.[7]

Men could argue that they are not asserting their own rights in the situation but are trying to protect the rights of the fetus. One feminist argument states that showing men as more sensitive to the rights or needs of the fetus impairs the image of the woman as sensitive because she is willing to abort the fetus. This 'feminizes' the man by giving him characteristics normally ascribed to women, and 'masculinizes' the woman by ascribing to her the qualities normally associated with men.[8] Is this fair? It hinges on gender essentialism – that men and women are different by virtue of their biological sex. This is obvious on the surface. Taken to a greater depth, the argument of feminization of the male assumes men cannot be sensitive to the needs of fetuses and children because this is essentially a female characteristic. There is no proof to support this, any more than there is proof to support claims that women cannot have so-called masculine characteristics by virtue of their female biology. However, there is sociological and psychological proof to indicate that men and women are socialized differently and therefore reason differently and respond differently in similar situations.[9]

More important than the essentialism of the above debate is the truth that it is the woman who will experience the physical burden of the pregnancy and the risks it involves. As a result, any interests in the rights of the father or the fetus would have to challenge the woman's right to choose whether or not she wishes to take these risks.

Bodily integrity: is it inviolable?

Bodily integrity considers the dangers and burdens of pregnancy, but it goes beyond this. The notion of bodily integrity incorporates recognition of the subjectivity of the individual. To use poetic language, it is respect for the 'I' that is embodied, the self, the ghost in the machine. The body is generally protected in law as inviolable, e.g. the right to refuse to supply blood or DNA samples for police investigation, the right to refuse to provide life-sustaining bone marrow or kidney donations. However, cases indicate that the body has not been treated as inviolable in pregnant women.[10] Occasional cases of forced caesarean sections and nonvoluntary sterilization (especially of disabled and poor women) suggest that this is the case. Is it a contradiction in our culture? Further examples show that pregnant women risk being treated as mere living incubators. This is shown most clearly in cases where elective ventilation has been used on pregnant women to bring infants to viability. Women tend to be expected to efface their own autonomy, desires and wishes in favour of the fetus.[11] Many women do this voluntarily and gladly to protect their unborn children. However, it is not just because of fetal rights that they do this. Can the mother's right to bodily integrity ever take primacy in abortion cases?

Women can be said to have the right to do as they wish with their own bodies. The section on informed consent (Chapter 3, p. 52) explains how any unauthorized touching, even for medical purposes, is equivalent to assault or battery. This is based on respect for bodily integrity. Thus women have been given the right to terminate pregnancies because the pregnancies affect their bodies, even though it is clear that this overrides the right or potential rights of the fetus. Most women will willingly consent to the risks of pregnancy and even, nowadays, intrauterine treatment of the fetus, if this is required. Bodily integrity is of little interest to many in most cases.

Special cases?

It is possible to take a middle of the road position about abortion and say that it is acceptable only in certain cases. A consequentialist, for example, might permit an abortion where harm will come to the mother if the pregnancy continues or when the fetus is diagnosed as being severely disabled. This is reflected in British law about abortion that permits therapeutic abortion in cases where physical or psychological harm is likely to befall the woman involved or when having another child will interfere with the interests of living children under her care. British law also permits therapeutic termination of pregnancy when the child is affected by severe disabilities. The question becomes one of measuring harm and, again, in the UK under the Abortion Act (1967), this is left to the discretion of the doctor, provided a second doctor witnesses an agreement.[12] Psychological harm is more difficult to determine than physical harm. It is uncertain whether it constitutes an abuse of the law to permit an abortion for social rather than physical reasons.

- Mrs K was concerned for her family's welfare because she felt she would be unable to handle the extra financial and emotional stress of a fifth child. Would this have been sufficient reason to permit the abortion?
- She then added that she had considered self-harm and suicide. Does this make an abortion more acceptable?

Under British laws as they currently stand, either of these reasons would be sufficient, on its own, because they indicate psychological distress and concern for the interests of existing viable children. Other cases where abortion has been considered acceptable by some is when the pregnancy is the result of rape or incest. In all these cases it is the consideration of harm that is used to justify the termination of pregnancy. Either because of potential harm to the mother or because of a harm already committed that no one wants to perpetuate.

Other social reasons that might be given are often finance- or career-related. Here the responsibility might focus on general social institutions and raise questions about why a woman may feel she needs to terminate a pregnancy because she cannot afford to have a child or to protect her chances of career advancement. Resolving this dilemma will require a look at a wider social responsibility.

Further considerations are made in this respect as well. The age and level and competence of the mother often constitute special cases for reservations against abortion. In the UK, girls under the age of 16 do not require parental permission to undergo an abortion if they are considered Gillick competent (see Chapter 2, p. 26). This means that a girl under the age of 16 can consent to an abortion provided a doctor has sufficient cause to believe that she is competent to make the decision on her own, and that she is able to understand her options and the potential consequences and risks involved.[13]

In the past, mentally disabled women were sometimes forced to have abortions and submit to sterilization for paternalistic reasons, i.e. what was perceived as being in their own best interests. Lately, this has come to be regarded as a violation and, more recently, families and custodians have had to seek legal permission to carry this out.

Case 29
Involuntary sterilization of an incapacitated teenager

Ms J is a 16-year-old girl who suffers from severe physical and mental disabilities and is unable to vocalize at all. She does seem to have some degree of understanding and communicates slightly through facial expression and hand gesticulations. Ms J is confined to a special wheelchair and is completely unable to care for herself regarding dressing, eating, personal hygiene, etc. and so requires 24-hour care. She has no other significant medical history but for the past 2 years has suffered from moderate menstrual pain and very heavy periods.

Ms J is a resident of a nursing home because her parents are in poor health, but she often stays with them at weekends. The patient's mother is worried that her daughter might be exploited, resulting in a pregnancy and that, because her daughter would be unable to care for the child, the responsibility would fall on her. There have been no problems of this nature at the home in the past but the mother has read about several such incidents in the media and is concerned for her daughter's welfare. She asks about the possibilities of having her daughter sterilized, and what other options are available to her.

After discussion about the clinical and legal aspects of the mother's request, it was agreed between the mother and the consultant to start the patient on regular Depo-Provera injections both to treat her painful and heavy periods and to address her mother's concerns regarding contraception.[14]

A set of helpful 'factors which could enable us to arrive at an ethically justifiable method of making a medical decision' in this context has been published.[15] These distinguish two major criteria and six minor criteria for consideration before a decision can be arrived at regarding the sterilization of a woman with incapacities who is of childbearing potential. The major criteria are heredity (regarding the likelihood of passing on similar disabilities to their offspring) and parenting competence. Once these have been addressed satisfactorily and sterilization is not determined to be necessary on either account, the six minor criteria must also be debated. These are:

1. conception risk
2. IQ
3. age
4. personality
5. medical aspects and prognosis
6. support and guidance for the mentally handicapped person.

The concern must always be founded upon the interests of the patient and not the ease or discomfort of society. As the authors of this set of useful criteria have put it:

Ultimately it comes down to deciding whether the benefits of sterilisation outweigh the drawbacks and whether the means are appropriate to the end, where efficient contraception is the end and irreversible sterilisation is the means.[16]

The result of such an analysis of Ms J's case would probably reveal the necessity of some form of contraception because she could not be a competent parent, nor would she be likely to be able to give valid consent to a pregnancy. Even so, there are clinical concerns about the effects the surgery and anaesthetic could have on Ms J, so a deeply invasive treatment of the sort involved in sterilization would probably not be in her best interest. Moreover, the first of the six minor conditions was dubious under the circumstances. The risk of her being raped in the home was a remote possibility, but adequate security arrangements would have been a more suitable response than invasive medical treatment. In the event, a suitable conclusion was reached on the basis of clinically warranted treatment for her menstrual symptoms that truly did benefit Ms J, and also provided reassurance about contraception.

Selective abortion in multiple pregnancies

Another circumstance in which abortion might be considered permissible is when a woman may be carrying multiple fetuses. In extreme cases when a woman has conceived as many as eight or nine babies at one time there will be concern for the pregnancy, the mother and the potential viable babies. In the UK this was made painfully real in the following case study.

Case 30
Selective abortion[17]

The tale of Mandy Allwood, a 31-year-old woman pregnant with eight fetuses, hit the headlines when her boyfriend released it to a

Birmingham news agency. Their exclusive story appeared in the *News of the World*, which had agreed to pay a reputed £100 000 provided that she has eight, or nearly eight, live babies.

Ms Allwood, who was having fertility treatment at a private clinic in the Midlands, was given urofollitrophin and chorionic gonadotrophin and warned not to have sexual intercourse after she superovulated, a warning she ignored. Questions were raised as to why she was having the treatment when she not only had one child aged 5 but had subsequently had an abortion and a miscarriage. Her boyfriend, Paul Hudson, did not live with her and spent several nights a week with his other girlfriend, with whom he had two children.

Ms Allwood was referred to Professor Nicolaides, a leading expert on selective reduction, who advised her to have the number of fetuses reduced to two. But she decided to try to deliver all eight babies.

Professor Nicolaides said: 'There is a great risk that she will just miscarry. The only hope is that she will get to 26–30 weeks and then hopefully some of the babies will survive. But there will be a risk of handicap from prematurity. All of the complications of pregnancy are exponentially increased with an increasing number of foetuses.'[16]

Sadly, all eight babies were stillborn at 19 weeks.

Not all multiple pregnancies will end in tragedy like this one. In fact, just months after this case was reported, an American woman delivered most of the babies from her multiple pregnancy alive. Nevertheless, the high risk of miscarriage of all fetuses makes an arguably strong justification for selective termination of some fetuses.[18] Unfortunately, the technique itself is risky and can cause miscarriage. Moreover, only fetuses that can be accessed easily will be aborted and this could mean that healthy fetuses are terminated whereas less healthy ones will live, only to miscarry later on in the pregnancy or die a few days after birth. But the hardest ethical question is whether it is acceptable to take the life of one potentially viable fetus to protect the life of another? And in cases where the multiple pregnancy means just two babies are being carried, can selective termination ever be justified as therapeutic?

Double effect: is it hypocrisy?

Situations in which abortion is used for therapeutic reasons often rely on the doctrine of the double effect to justify the termination. This:

> Permits an act which is foreseen to have both good and bad effects provided: the act itself is good or at least indifferent; the good effect is the reason for acting; the good effect is not caused by the bad effect; a proportionate reason exists for causing the bad effect, e.g. morphine for pain may shorten a life.[19]

According to this doctrine, abortion could be justified if it were *intended* as a therapeutic measure to treat the mother. This need not be a life-or-death situation for the mother, but could also be intended to ease her physical, psychological or emotional distress. Abortion for reasons of genetic abnormality is usually considered here as well. This will be discussed in greater detail below.

Doctors' duties

Doctors are permitted to be conscientious objectors to abortion; however, it is the duty of the doctor to inform the patient of her options and to offer to refer her to someone who will carry out the abortion. Because abortion is a matter of conscience, no health-care professional should have to assist in an abortion except under emergency circumstances.[20] Unfortunately, recent literature suggests that doctors, whose rights of conscientious objection are generally recognized by their professional bodies, have been discriminated against for refusing to provide abortions themselves.[21] Such discrimination imposes unnecessary burdens upon those who are opposed to abortion to provide services when others can be found who are willing to do so.

Regardless of their position on abortion, doctors must be careful not to coerce the patient into accepting a particular choice. Because of the vulnerability of the patient, the doctor is in a situation of power and can be in a position to coerce a decision. This contradicts the respect for patient autonomy that is so cherished in contemporary medical practice.

The Abortion Act 1967 of England 'originally set no limit to the time when an abortion might lawfully be performed.'[22] However, protection of the health of the woman makes abortion past 24 weeks clinically inadvisable and this is recognized in the law. Therapeutic abortions where the child is considered to have severe congenital abnormalities, such as anencephaly, are permitted under the Act at any time during the pregnancy.

Childbirth

Closely related to the debate about abortion is the debate about the mother's freedom to control childbirth. The process of childbirth has become medicalized over the centuries. For many women it is no longer a matter of home births and natural labour. Instead technology has overtaken the birthing process, and with very good reason, because this has reduced many of the risks of childbirth and improved the chances of having a healthy mother and child at the end of the process. These improvements have brought with them restrictions to the choices women can make but have also given greater power to the medical establishment to reject those decisions women do make. This is usually justified on the grounds that women are not capable of rational consideration of the options while they are in the throes of labour. This is a position that has been challenged convincingly in debates over cases in which women have been forced to have caesarean sections against their wishes. To try to avoid such incidents, many countries advocate the use of birthplans. These permit women to consider in advance what their choices might be given possible eventualities. So women can choose what sort of pain control they wish to use, if any, whether and when they want to be induced if they pass their due date, and other relevant decisions. These plans are discussed with midwives and obstetricians and are supposed to be followed unless the woman herself authorizes a change.

In situations during labour where women are confronted with an unexpected turn of events that typically suggests invasive techniques, such as forceps delivery or caesarean section, dubious challenges to their birthplans can occur. On occasions, women have been forced to undergo these invasive procedures, even when they have discussed their refusal in advance and have strong reasons for wanting to reject these invasions of their bodily integrity.[23] More often than not, women in the middle of difficult labour will take all available help, especially in emergency situations. Few women are likely to refuse emergency treatment to save the life of their child or even their own lives. In rare cases, however, some women have refused emergency care, and here healthcare professionals and judges usually challenge their decisions. Cases of forced caesarean sections appear in the legal literature. These take the form of debate about the competence of women during labour. This should hopefully be avoided by prior discussion of birthplans. But in situations where the woman is asked to defend her position in the midst of medical crisis, it is hard to say who is not reasoning clearly, the woman or those who expect her to defend her choice during the throes of labour.

Once again, this calls into question the idea of bodily integrity. In most other contexts, enforced treatment is considered an assault. Here, the reasons in favour of it tend to include the apparent contradiction implied if a woman willingly carries a child to term and then refuses to undergo treatment that will save the child's life. This could be true of a woman who suddenly makes the choice or makes it on the basis of irrational fears. But unless a flaw in her reasoning can be found, the reasons she offers might be compelling enough to make them acceptable, even if we find it hard to agree with them. This is especially true of reasons based upon long-standing deep commitments, such as religious belief. Simply because we as doctors disagree with a decision does not necessarily mean that the decision is wrong. More discussion of this last topic can be found in Chapter 2 (p. 33) and Chapter 3 (p. 61).

Infertility and assisted reproduction

Involuntary childlessness is less of a problem than it used to be. There are many opportunities now available to assist subfertile women and men to have children. Techniques range from high-tech ones such as *in vitro* fertilization (IVF), gamete intra fallopian transfer (GIFT) and cloning. Low-tech options usually include artificial insemination (AI), sometimes described in more emotive language as the 'virgin birth' technique, surrogate motherhood and adoption. This means that people who were unable to become parents in the past are more likely to be able to produce genetically related offspring. More recent techniques have also been used to ensure that the children we give birth to approximate the kind of children we want.

People suffering from infertility, postmenopausal women, gay and lesbian couples and single parents are among the new range of parental hopefuls. Cases reported in the media have raised scandals when supposed concern for the unborn children has permitted public intrusion into the private choices of individuals. There have been accusations of selfishness among those who want children but are not able to have them naturally and seek funded medical treatment to do so. It is not clear whether or when it is appropriate for otherwise private choices to be restricted in deference to public concerns, but the debate emerges in several aspects related to the technology of human reproduction and genetic manipulation.

Screening and genetics

Many new possibilities arose at the end of the twentieth century for couples who wish to control conception, and even the characteristics of their children. In this section we will cover the following issues, using a mixture of true and invented cases as illustrations.

- Antenatal screening
- Preimplantation screening: therapeutic and elective
- Genetic manipulation, 'designer babies' and discrimination
- Cloning.

Antenatal screening

Case 31
Antenatal screening

Lorna, 37 and Gus, 38 have been married for 3 years and are overjoyed when Lorna finally becomes pregnant. Lorna was adopted herself and feels strongly about the importance of family. They are eager to become parents but are realistic about the dramatic life-changes parenthood will have, so they agree to undergo antenatal screening and testing if it becomes necessary, 'just to be sure we know what to expect' says Lorna. The couple recognizes their freedom to have a therapeutic termination of pregnancy if the results are positive and they tell their doctor that they are open to the possibility.

Antenatal screening has appeared as a blessing for many families who have entered parenthood with the foreknowledge that they are likely to be raising a child with a particular genetic condition such as Down syndrome or spina bifida. It has also given these families the opportunity to terminate fetuses affected with similar conditions, and screening programmes are often described as attempts to reduce costs and hardships by eliminating the conditions altogether. As public health strategies, screening programmes are justified on largely utilitarian grounds. The benefits of reduced hardship and costs of care are found to outweigh any potential harms. Here we will examine some of the potential benefits and costs that accompany antenatal screening and testing.

Benefits
The greatest benefit cited by most proponents of antenatal screening is the greater freedom of choice it affords us to decide whether or not to introduce into the world children who will live with apparently burdensome conditions that could severely affect the quality of their lives. Added to this are the reduced risks to mothers carrying affected fetuses for which they may endure difficult labours or miscarriages.

The most obvious and wide-ranging advantages of screening programmes come to the population in general. Reduced costs of care, which are usually high related to the conditions screened for, means that funding could be channelled into other areas of healthcare. Put simply, the population as a whole benefits when there is a reduction in births of children who require costly and lengthy healthcare treatment. Most of us tend to, and perhaps prefer to, ignore this final long-term benefit because it combines with the distasteful implication that we choose to save money rather than look after those who need it most. However, this utilitarian advantage is real and does help to justify screening and termination in some cases. It should not be overlooked, though, that the reasons are more often related to the benefits and protection from hardships

of the children and the families involved. The economic advantage is not the reason screening tests were invented in the first place, rather it is more likely that they were created with a deontological aim of reducing suffering and helping those involved.

Problems
Despite the good intentions and the many benefits of screening and testing, there are some significant harms as well. Chief among these is the worry and concern attached to antenatal screening for most women who undergo the procedure, and especially for those who are found to have high likelihood of carrying an affected child. In some cases these will be false positives and the woman will continue to worry unnecessarily. The risks do not stop with the screening. Positive screening is not the same as a diagnosis and most women who screen positive will then undergo amniocentesis, which is uncomfortable and carries with it a 0.5% risk of causing spontaneous miscarriage even in healthy pregnancies.

Other concerns include further social stratification implied by value judgements in screening for certain conditions. Does screening for a particular condition mean that we devalue those who are eventually born with it? Some women have reported feeling pressured to choose a termination of pregnancy in cases where the child is diagnosed with the condition. It might be that institutionalized screening eliminates real choice for parents to decide to carry on such pregnancies or refuse to participate in screening in the first place.

It is often explicitly assumed that 'reproductive choice' will mean that parents will decide to abort fetuses found to have genetic disorders, but if we are to take the concepts of choice and autonomy seriously we have to allow for the possibility of parents deciding to carry an affected fetus to term. One concern is that this choice will increasingly be eroded by pressures, including those from insurance companies, to abort.[24]

List reasons why you agree or disagree with the following statements:

- Antenatal genetic screening can support individual liberties and social values

- Antenatal genetic screening can erode individual liberties and social values

---

Preimplantation screening

Where the screening is for mild conditions it is difficult to know what will be permissible. The line might seem less blurred where the suffering related to the condition is more defined.[25] In these cases there is little doubt that parents have a right to go into the choice knowledgeably and with the liberty to choose one way or the other. Consider the following development in Lorna and Gus's case and the options made available to them.

Case 31 continued
Therapeutic preimplantation screening

As events unfold, the screening test indicates no cause for concern that Lorna and Gus's baby will be affected by Down syndrome or spina bifida and, in due course, Lorna gives birth to a son, Charlie.

They live in sleepless bliss for 3 years. Then, just as the couple is considering a second

---

pregnancy, Charlie begins to show signs that something is wrong. He is eventually diagnosed with Duchenne muscular dystrophy. As it turns out, Lorna, unbeknownst to her, is a carrier of this disease, which is passed on maternally even though the woman will be unaffected herself, i.e. it is a disease that affects only males. The family is distraught at the prospect of Charlie's suffering and eventual untimely death.

While they are adjusting to the reality of their circumstance, a genetic counsellor suggests that the couple would be eligible for preimplantation screening for future pregnancies. This is a process in which, as a minimum, the sex of embryos, and sometimes the genetic condition itself, can be determined following *in vitro* fertilization (IVF). It has the aim of ensuring that only healthy embryos are implanted. In this case, only female embryos would be implanted to prevent Lorna and Gus having a second son with this devastating illness.

Gus says, 'we wouldn't give up our son for anything, and we know there is no certainty in this world, but to be able to have a child who we know wouldn't have to suffer as Charlie is would really mean the world to us.'

This takes the freedom to choose a step further. The ability to determine the sex or genetic make-up of a child prior to implantation certainly is seen to have some advantages over antenatal screening and testing.

> …because genetic tests before implantation can remove the need for abortion they are a preferred approach for couples who are offered the choice.[26]

Consider why a person might agree and disagree with the preceding quote.

There are significant advantages to preimplantation diagnosis because it involves far less danger to the mother, who will not have to endure the physical risks of a termination. But the procedure does leave open the question, what is the moral status of discarded embryos? Some of the embryos will be retained and others will not. In Lorna and Gus's case only female fetuses with no chance of developing the disease will be retained. What ought to happen to the male fetuses? The question is certainly still up for debate, but there are at least three possibilities.

1. They can be disposed of as other living tissue is in the medical context. This might seem callous to some, but at least they can be given a ceremonious disposal and permit the parents to end their commitment to them.
2. They can be retained and used for treatment or scientific research. Stem cell treatment and other forms of scientific advances have been performed using aborted or discarded fetal tissue to great success. The advantage to this solution is that whatever loss is felt in the decision not to implant fetuses for pregnancy, it is perhaps balanced by a sense that some good will result. Nevertheless, there is wide objection on moral grounds to the use of fetal tissue in experimentation. People are often repulsed by the idea, especially where pregnancy and abortion might be instigated specifically for the purpose of research or treatment.[27] However, in Lorna and Gus's case the fetuses were not created for that express purpose but were deselected by the parents for therapeutic reasons. They can be of some help to others. Is this option any more problematic than merely discarding them?
3. The third, less commonly considered option, is to offer the embryos to other couples who cannot produce embryos of their own. This is an odd kind of adoption where the biological parents give up the responsibility and care for potential children and either the adoptive mother or a surrogate mother carries the child to term. This can create a new set of problems. What if a child is born who is not affected by the condition? Can the biological

parents change their minds and retrieve the child within a given period of time? Must the adoptive parents know about the possible genetic condition carried by the child? Is it a better option than ordinary abortion or the two possibilities discussed above? Do we have an obligation to implant all embryos? What if no suitable mother can be found?

Whichever option is chosen, the initial problem is the discarding of potentially healthy fetuses. Lorna and Gus have clinically justifiable reasons for this, but what if they didn't?

Genetic manipulation and non-therapeutic screening

Case 32
Tragic couple mount battle to choose sex of test tube baby[28]

A grieving couple whose only daughter was killed in a bonfire accident last year have launched a historic battle to win the right to choose the sex of their next child.

Alan and Louise Masterton, from Monifieth, in Angus, will attempt to force doctors to implant her with female-only embryos, a request that would mean any male embryos would have to be destroyed.

The Health and Fertilisation Authority (HFEA), which regulates infertility clinics, has already turned down the couple's plea for a change in the law, but they said last night they were determined to fight on.

Louise, who was sterilized after giving birth to Nicole 3 years ago, insists that she is not trying to replace their daughter.

'We don't want a designer baby and we are not trying to replace Nicky,' she said. 'We just want the chance to make our family whole again'.

The couple, both aged 42, have four sons aged from 15 to 9 and have warned that they are prepared to travel abroad to have the operation if the guidelines are not changed in Britain.

'We know another girl won't replace Nicky but we want the chance to try,' [Alan said]. 'We don't think choice of sex should be there for everybody but we are not everybody. What has happened to us is thankfully very, very rare. The technology exists for us to have a baby girl and we want to use it. Is that so wrong?'

The couple is now embroiled in a battle against the HFEA, to gain permission to sex screen their test tube baby.

But the authority is resisting any change to the rule that bestows that choice only on prospective parents who are carriers of gender-specific medical conditions.

The Mastertons have already won the support of a range of medical ethics lawyers, psychologists and doctors, as well as their local MP, Andrew Welsh, who is to raise the matter in Westminster.

A dossier on the couple's case was submitted to the HFEA executive a few weeks ago but the organization has refused to comment.

This leaves us brimming with questions. How much should we be allowed to determine the genetic inheritance of our children? Is it wise to let parents make genetic choices affecting a child's sex? height? IQ? sexual orientation?[29] Some of these choices are possible now. Others could become so in the near future.[30] We do recognize the rights of parents to do what they think will protect or further their children's best interests. We make no argument against permitting parents to choose whether or not to vaccinate their child, to select schools and raise their children in specific social or religious contexts. So why not permit them to select those attributes they think will be best for their child?

The most likely responses to this are based on concerns about natural distribution of genetic characteristics and a concern for maintaining a balance that resembles that of nature. Permitting parents to choose the sex of their children could lead to over selection of one sex or another as social trends change. Furthermore, genetic traits are neither good nor bad in themselves but only in the way they are socially valued. Thus it is neither better nor worse to have a certain skin or eye colour, it is only preferred or rejected because of social preference, stigma and prejudice. These are value judgements and ought to be resolved not by eliminating the least favoured characteristics but by eliminating the prejudice that devalues them.

Parents might respond that they have suffered in ways they hope to protect their children from suffering, namely prejudice and stigma related to characteristics irrelevant to their abilities to contribute to their communities. They will say they have suffered enough and ought to be permitted to give their children the best possible advantages even if it reinforces negative stereotypes. These arguments would be difficult to contradict. All we can do is try to eliminate the prejudicial attitudes that reinforce their perception.

Finally, permitting genetic selection and manipulation for non-therapeutic advantages will not actually solve any problems in the long run, it will merely move the territory in which they apply. The same could even be true for therapeutic selection. Currently we might seek to remove genes for disabling conditions such as severe spina bifida or Down syndrome; eventually we could seek to change less disabling conditions such as susceptibility to colds in order to reduce loss of income due to sick days. The problem is that there will always be some genetic characteristic believed to be less valuable than another. Eventually, we might sink towards the terrifying future of Aldous Huxley's *Brave New World*, where there are few genetic differences such that sameness is valued more highly than that which makes us unique. Clinically, there is no telling what potentially devastating system we could be setting up, where lack of genetic differentiation makes us susceptible to lethal organisms that might have been relatively less destructive had there been a greater variety of genetic composition to combat them.

Having said all this, we are still left with the desirability of at least some genetic manipulation to promote characteristics that make us less susceptible to the ravages of disease and the painful losses that accompany them.

Cloning[31]

What if we take the Mastertons' story a little bit further and into the realm of science fiction?

Case 32 continued
Cloning around

Imagine a future scenario where a couple in a similar circumstance to the Mastertons discovers that samples of their daughter's DNA are being stored at the hospital where she died. The parents apply to retrieve some of the DNA in order to produce an embryo clone for implantation, effectively creating an identical twin of their lost daughter. Should they be permitted to do this?

As this book is being written, news headlines abound declaring that a human being will be cloned in the next 12 months. There is no telling whether this will happen or not. However, the technology does seem to be present and, if this is so, then the actuality of human cloning is likely too. Questions about the ethics of research are addressed elsewhere in this book (see Chapter 7). This section seeks to examine positions relative to the acceptability of human cloning as a treatment policy. Should we clone human beings? What do we gain or lose from cloning? Would it constitute a threat to the right of individuality? How would it affect the rights of parents versus those of the children produced?[32]

Our gut instinct to the case under discussion is to reject the parents' wishes as the

stuff of horror movies, but why? The main concern seems to be that the child will suffer undue pressure to be just like the donor child. Every child deserves to be valued for his or her unique gifts. Cloning in this case could allow the parents to ignore the child's individual worth. It also reduces the value of the first child to imagine her to be replaceable or recreated. If you lose one child, can you simply go back and make another? Or is something lost that was inherently unique and that can never be found again? There can be no worse loss for the parents, but creating a clone of the child is not going to ease their loss.

Scientific advances in cloning technology have dispelled the likelihood of a science fiction expectation that one could clone an exact replica of a particular person. We know from the experience of Dolly the sheep, cloned at the Roslin Institute in Scotland, that the clone will have a different independent existence, even if it is genetically identical to the donor of the genetic material. The same is true of identical twins in nature. Reports of uncanny similarities aside, identical twins live different lives and experience different things despite their identical makeup. This is because, although they are called identical, the identity is not the one-to-one identity of mathematics, so they will be different in some respects. It follows for clones too. They will be alike but, because it is impossible to reproduce the exact set of experiences that contribute to their upbringing and narrative development, the clones cannot be identical to their original donor.

This might ease our concerns related to the individuality of particular persons. We can protect this by the assurance that their lives will be different and that therefore their narrative identities will be too. Of greater concern is the protection of genetic diversity, already suggested in this chapter to be essential for protection from disease. Is it acceptable to copy entire races of human beings? The response to this must be 'no', because it is clinically unjustifiable to reject genetic diversity. Any advantages of genetic identity across the world, such as an end to racial prejudice, would be overruled by the danger that a single disease could destroy the human race entirely.

Cloning will be better used as medical treatment. The possibility of cloning organs instead of entire humans has been foreshadowed and would have real benefits for organ implantation. First, fewer people would require donor organs, because they could be implanted with a heart, liver or kidney grown especially for them. The added advantage that the cloned organ would be less likely to be rejected makes the process even more desirable. Other therapeutic uses of cloning technology are found in treatment for infertility. A couple could use their own genetic material to create an embryo through IVF. The embryo could then be implanted in the genetic mother or in a surrogate mother and carried to term. The clear advantage to this is that the child would be the genetic offspring of the eventual legal or nurturing parents, unlike situations where the child is adopted or the result of donated egg, sperm or both. These therapeutic uses of cloning technology have strong benefits. The use of cloning intended by our fictional case couple is more dubious. Can one be allowed and not the other?

> On the basis of this discussion about the ethical challenges presented by genetics, what proposals could be made to ensure genetics is applied responsibly in new reproductive technologies?

Surrogacy

The most low-tech treatment for infertility is surrogacy. A woman can offer to carry a child to term to help a couple who are having trouble doing so on their own. The understanding is that, after the delivery, the child will be given to the couple who sought

the help and the surrogate will have no responsibility to the new child or its family. Despite the relative simplicity of surrogacy compared to other technologies, problems abound:

- Concern for the psychological and physical health of the surrogate mother
- Concern for the psychological and physical health of the children
- Concern for the psychological health of the adoptive parents
- Concern for society and social institutions
- Problems of compliance.

The most famous case regarding surrogacy occurred in the US in the mid-1980s.

Case 33
Baby M[33]

Mary Beth Whitehead was contracted to act as a surrogate mother and was also the genetic mother of the baby she was carrying for William and Elizabeth Stern; William Stern was the genetic father through artificial insemination. Mr Stern contracted with Mrs Whitehead for her to be the surrogate mother for the Sterns' child; in return, they promised to pay her $10 000 and to pay her medical expenses. Several days after the birth, she asked the Sterns to allow her to take the baby home for a week; the Sterns agreed. The next day, Mrs Whitehead left the state to visit her mother. Shortly thereafter, Mrs Whitehead told the Sterns that she wanted to keep the baby and she eluded a subsequent court order requiring her to return the baby to the Sterns. She ran away with the baby for almost 3 months. After numerous press conferences, suits and countersuits, the court awarded custody of the baby to the Sterns but gave Mrs Whitehead visitation rights. However, the court did not uphold the enforceability of the surrogacy contract itself; rather, it awarded custody on the basis of what it considers to be 'the best interests of the child'.

The public reaction to the case of Baby M was both deep and widespread. Many sympathized with Mrs Whitehead and decried the action of the court as taking a child from her 'real' mother. Others sympathized with the Sterns, who had placed their trust and hopes for a family with Mrs Whitehead. They saw Mrs Whitehead's promise to the Sterns as binding. Some sympathized with both sides, as well as with the baby, and denounced the situation itself, calling for the banning of all surrogacy arrangements precisely because they could lead to such Solomonic outcomes.

In the past, couples who preferred to try adoption through a surrogate mother would find a suitable and willing candidate who would, like Mary Beth Whitehead, voluntarily be impregnated via artificial insemination (AI), preferably with sperm from the intending father. After the delivery, the parents of the child would be the biological parents, namely the surrogate mother and the donating father. The father's wife or partner would then legally adopt the child and the surrogate/biological mother would end her relationship with the child and adoptive couple. Problems arise when the surrogate mother refuses to uphold the prior agreement and decides to keep the child. The law was originally quite clear on the matter. In ordinary cases of divorce, for example, it was usually considered to be in the best interests of the child to be left with the mother. And where the man applying for adoptive status was not the biological father, but instead the child was the product of AI using donor sperm, the custody of the child was not even really in question from a legal point of view. However, in cases where a surrogacy contract had been the intended origin of the pregnancy, it was no longer obvious how the interests of the child would be best served. More often than not the adoptive family was more wealthy or stable and in a traditionally better position to provide for the child. The surrogate mother in some cases agreed to the pregnancy because she needed the money that came with it.

It was on this account that the law determined early on that money ought not to be part of the agreement. Many reasons are offered for this. Prime among them is the fear of degrading the value of the child by turning him or her into a commodity. The same argument can be extended to the surrogate mother, whose womb should not be reduced to a mere consumer item. A further argument was added that women might be exploited if they were enticed to act as surrogates, with the accompanying risks of pregnancy, for the sake of the money. None of these possibilities appears palatable. As a result, many countries restrict the amount of money offered a woman to act as a surrogate to the costs incurred by her to ensure a safe and healthy pregnancy.[34] This will include medical costs and sometimes rent, food and clothing if it is required. No additional fee will be paid, despite the added risk to her health, the time required (including time off from work) or the potential hardships involved. In the US, where there is precedence for sales in the medical context, such as sale of blood, the regulations against payment are far more relaxed. This at least acknowledges the risks and effort involved for the woman who agrees to act as a surrogate but it leaves intact the concern about reducing human beings to consumer goods.

The issue grows more complicated when, like Mary Beth Whitehead, the surrogate mother changes her mind about the agreement. In the case of Baby M, Mrs Whitehead was the biological mother. So it was her conflict with the biological father, Mr Stern, and the contract between Whitehead and the Sterns, that caused the case to come to public attention. If Baby M had been the product of both donor sperm and egg, or an embryo created by IVF from the cultivated egg and sperm of the Sterns', the situation would have been far more complex. And this is the stage of complexity that technology has now reached. Lawrence Hinman has created an instructive table (Table 8.1) that helps clarify the possibilities to an extent. He calls it 'the vocabulary of the new parenthood'.[35]

Table 8.1
The vocabulary of new parenthood[35]

Stakeholder	Description
Intentional mother	The woman who wants to have the child
Intentional father	The man who wants to have the child
Genetic mother	The woman who supplies the egg for the embryo
Genetic father	The man who supplies the sperm for the embryo
Gestational mother	The woman who carries the embryo to term and gives birth to it
Nurturing mother	The woman who raises and nurtures the child from infancy as her own
Nurturing father	The man who raises and nurtures the child from infancy as his own

Under Hinman's vocabulary there are multiple possible stakeholders in the creation of a child, many of whom exist only because of new technologies. We cannot yet begin to determine what degree of commitment is owed to any of these stakeholders, let alone how much responsibility they owe the offspring of the complicated relationships. For example, what is the relationship between the gestational mother and child if the child is the product of a donor egg? What is clear is that each of these 'parents' has an interest in whatever relationship they eventually have with the child and the possibility for exploitation of human beings is great. So far, there is no clear way of avoiding the exploitation, but the laws of different countries have tried. Removing the financial aspect of the contracts has been a first choice in the UK. This eases the distaste of buying and selling babies and wombs, but forces the surrogate mother and the women who donate eggs to undergo risky, onerous procedures and processes as acts of charity and altruism without being rewarded for it financially. So the allegations of exploitation of women still

exist, although, as we saw above, the arguments concerning exploitation are equally strong if surrogate mothers are paid.

The advantages of surrogacy still remain. It is low-tech in some circumstances and offers solutions to women who are unable to sustain a pregnancy. What is amazing is that in an age of high-tech procedures, such as egg harvesting and IVF, the child of a surrogacy agreement can be the genetic offspring of the couple who raise it even if it bears no genetic relation to the gestational mother.

Conclusions

Although many issues have been addressed in this chapter, we have still not exhausted the ethical and legal problems related to human reproduction. As technological advances continue to increase our options, it looks as if we will need to continue to ask the questions and look for more and more answers. In this chapter we examined a few of the issues that raise the ethical problems in debate for many of the related topics:

- the rights of women
- the rights of men
- the rights of children
- social concerns
- natural concerns.

Throughout the chapter we have raised concerns for individuals and balanced these with concerns that society might have in the choices these individuals made or were allowed to make. We end with a quote from Michael Parker, which illustrates how human reproductive choices, especially those involving genetic manipulation, are on a narrow divide between private and public:

When, for example, are my reproductive choices, if ever, a matter for me and my family alone, to be made in the privacy of our own home, and when are they, again if ever, a matter for public decision making? In some ways genetics, especially when combined with new reproductive technology, seems to bring the private into the public arena.[36]

Notes and references

1 Brazier M. Medicine, patients and the law. Middlesex: Penguin Books; 1992:311.

2 Thomas JE, Waluchow WJ. Well and good: case studies in biomedical ethics, revised edn. Peterborough, Ontario: Broadview Press; 1990:49–53.

3 The most famous of these are works by the Princeton-based philosopher Peter Singer.

4 Jarvis-Thomson J. A defence of abortion. Philosophy and Public Affairs 1971; 1(1):47–66. Reprinted in Jarvis-Thomson J. Rights, restitution and risks: essays in moral theory. Cambridge, MA: Harvard University Press; 1986.

5 Bordo S. Unbearable weights. Berkeley, CA: California University Press; 1993:71–97.

6 See, for example, the case of Chantal Daigle and Jean Guy Tremblay in Quebec, Canada, as reported in: Thomas JE, Waluchow WJ. Well and good: case studies in biomedical ethics, revised edn. Peterborough, Ontario: Broadview Press; 1990:54–57.

7 Brazier M. Medicine, patients and the law. Middlesex: Penguin Books; 1992:301.

8 Bordo S. Unbearable weights. California University Press; 1993:71–97.

9 Gilligan C. In a different voice. Boston, MA: Harvard University Press ; 1982.

10 See cases reported in: Brazier M. Medicine, patients and the law. Middlesex: Penguin Books; 1992:254–257.

11 See: Bordo S. Unbearable weights. California University Press; 1993 and Jarvis-Thomson J. A defence of abortion. Philosophy and Public Affairs 1971; 1(1):47–66, reprinted in Jarvis-Thomson J. Rights, restitution and risks: essays in moral theory. Cambridge, MA: Harvard University Press; 1986.

12 United Kingdom Abortion Act 1967. London: HMSO.

13 Brazier M. Medicine, patients and the law. Middlesex: Penguin Books; 1992.

14 Louden S. Unpublished material; 2001.

15 Denekens JP et al. Sterilisation of incompetent mentally handicapped persons: a model for decision making. J Medical Ethics 1999; 25(3):237–241.

16 Dyer C. Selective abortions hit the headlines. Br Med J 1996: 313:380.

17 Mason J, McCall Smith R. Law and medical ethics. 5th edn. London: Butterworths; 1999:77.

18 Human Fertilisation and Embryology Act 1990. London: HMSO. Available at: http://www.legislation.hmso.gov.uk/acts/acts 1990/ukpga_19900037_en_1

19 Boyd K et al. eds. The new dictionary of medical ethics. London: BMJ Publications; 1997:76.

20 Wicclair MR. Conscientious objection in medicine. Bioethics 2000; 14(3):205–227.

21 Jones C. Conscientious objection: a right to refuse. BMA News Review, September 1999:18–20.

22 Brazier M. Medicine, patients and the law. Middlesex: Penguin Books; 1992.

23 Draper H. Women, forced caesareans and antenatal responsibilities. J Medical Ethics 1996; 22:327–333.

24 MacIntyre S. Social and psychological issues associated with the new genetics. Phil Trans R Soc London B 1997; 352:1095–1101.

25 Draper H, Chadwick R. Beware! Preimplantation genetic diagnosis may solve some old problems but it also raises new ones. J Medical Ethics 1999; 25:114–120.

26 Raeburn JA. Preimplantation diagnosis raises a philosophical dilemma. Br Med J 1994; Vol 311 Page 540.

27 Mason J, McCall Smith R. Law and medical ethics. 5th edn. London: Butterworths; 1999:361.

28 Hill A. Tragic couple mount battle to choose sex of test tube baby. Scotland on Sunday. 12 March 2000:3.

29 Reiss MJ. The ethics of genetic research of intelligence. Bioethics 2000; 14(1):1–15.

30 Available from: http://www.dartmouth.edu/artsci/ethics-inst/application1.html#course

31 Gibbs N. Baby, it's you! and you, and you…Time Magazine 2001; Monday 12 February 2001. Available at: http://www.bma.org.uk/nrezine.nsf/ 820ae71b42dd1920802569200055e3f9/a39eacc3d74f58 e780256996004e8178?Open Document

32 Amer MS. Breaking the mold: human embryo cloning and its implications. UCLA Law Review 1996; 43(5):1659–1688.

33 Hinman LM. Reproductive technology and surrogacy: an introduction to the issues. Available: http://ethics.acusd.edu/Papers/Introduction%20to% 20Reproductive%20Technologies.html

34 See: Surrogacy Arrangements Act 1985. London: HMSO and The Human Fertilisation and Embryology Act 1990. London: HMSO. Available at: http://www.hmso.gov.uk/acts/summary/01990037

35 Hinman LM. Reproductive technology and surrogacy: an introduction to the issues. Available: http://ethics.acusd.edu/Papers/Introduction%20to% 20Reproductive%20Technologies.html

36 Parker M. Public deliberation and private choice in genetics and reproduction. J Medical Ethics 2000; 26:160–165.

9

Rationing and rationality: issues in scarce resource allocation

The word 'rationing' is derived from the Latin term *ratio*, which can be translated into English as 'rationality'. Hence the notion of rationing is in some sense related to the idea of rationalizing or bringing order to chaos.[1] The chaos in this context is the imbalance between the scarcity of health resources on the one hand and the needs of those attempting to access them on the other. Because so many people are trying to access such a diversity of limited resources, it makes sense that we try to apply order to the way in which supplies will be used and distributed. This is why we find ourselves setting priorities where resources are scarce, but does it necessarily mean deliberate exclusion or denial of services?[2]

Is rationing inevitable?

The opening paragraph to this chapter implies that rationing and deprivation are inevitable. Some arguments suggest this is so because resources will always fall short of meeting individual and community demands. Other arguments deny that rationing is inevitable and insist that all needs could be met if only policy and spending were redirected to meet healthcare requirements.[3] But then from where will the money be redirected? Education? Environmental protection? Social welfare? This will only cause deprivation in other areas, many of which are equally as important as healthcare and also contribute to good health. For example, environmental protection preserves clean water, which in turn helps to maintain the health of the community.[4]

Many people believe that collecting additional funds through taxes will help solve the problem but there is a general unwillingness to accept tax increases. Besides, we cannot know how much would be required and therefore cannot predict where we would draw the line at increases. In some ways, health budgets look like bottomless pits, prompting comments such as the following from the British Secretary of State for Health in 1999:

> The NHS – just like every other health system in the world, public or private – has never, or will never, provide all the care it might theoretically be possible to provide. That would probably be true even if the whole of the UK gross domestic product was spent on health care. So within our expanding health system there will always be choices to be made about the care to be provided.[5]

We cannot be certain this pessimistic scenario is a necessity; however, it has proven to be the case for most healthcare systems. Will there ever be enough money to fund the entire medical needs and wants of an ever-growing population driven by a technologically ever-advancing field? It is difficult to say. In any case, it is realistic and not defeatist to acknowledge the need to make sense of the way we use healthcare resources, regardless of whether or not they are finite. Our response must be to acknowledge the obligation to set priorities in a responsible manner and, if finiteness exists, to recognize the obligation it imposes upon us to ration in a justifiable way.

At any rate, there will be areas where rationing is necessary because they rely on more than just money. Cost is a legitimate concern for a healthcare system but equally valuable and equally scarce are resources such as organs, technology, beds and energy. Organ donation is an example of how rationing pertains to resources beyond just money. It relies on the few suitable organs made available at any given time. Decisions about allocation and deprivation become very real when 20 people are on a waiting list and only one heart is available for donation.

Justifiable rationing

If we can assume that rationing is inevitable, how can rationing decisions be made in an ethical and socially responsible fashion? The first step might be to clearly define priorities in healthcare. But this is not as easy as it sounds.

> List three areas you would consider to be priorities in healthcare:
>
> 1.
> 2.
> 3.
>
> Compare this list with another person's list. Why do you suppose there is agreement? Why do you suppose there is disagreement?

At present, although there have been attempts, no prescribed systematic priority-setting models have been agreed upon in the UK;[6] therefore we end up with rationing by default. Other countries have attempted to apply models for justifiable rationing and prioritizing, with varying degrees of success, and none has been perfected.[7] A remedy to the uncertainty that plagues prioritizing decisions would need to include considerations of the following questions:

> If rationing cannot be avoided:
> • How should priority decisions be made?
> • Who ought to make priority decisions?

The case described below will help illustrate the complex web of issues involved in rationing decisions and the emotional reactions that surface when rationing leads to deprivation for a particular person or group. Later in this chapter, a second case on flu medication will be used to illustrate broader considerations.

> ### Case 34
> ### Child B[8]
>
> *R. v. Cambridge Health Authority*, ex p B; Court of Appeal. [1995] 2 All ER 129, (1995) Times, 15 March
>
> B, a girl aged 10, had contracted non-Hodgkin's lymphoma with common acute lymphoblastic leukaemia at the age of five. Despite initially successful treatment, in 1993 she developed acute myeloid leukaemia. After further chemotherapy and an allogenic bone marrow transplant, the disease went into remission. However, in January 1995 she suffered a relapse. Doctors who had treated her considered that a further course of chemotherapy followed by a second transplant would not be in her best interests. They gave her 6–8 weeks to live and said that they could not treat her further.
>
> Her father applied to the hospital authority (to fund an experimental treatment). He found a doctor who was willing to offer further chemotherapy and, if that proved successful, a further transplant. As a bed was unavailable on the National Health Service, the treatment would have to be carried out privately. The chances of a complete remission following chemotherapy were assessed at around 10%, at a cost of £15 000; while the chances for the transplant, costing £60 000, which would be performed if the chemotherapy were completed successfully, were put in the same region. The authority declined the father's application to fund the treatment.
>
> B's father, as her next friend, applied for an order of certiorari quashing the authority's decision not to fund the treatment for her, and applied for an order of mandamus to direct the authority to fund the treatment.

Ordinarily, rationing decisions and scarce resource allocation take place in the anonymous context of public policy-making. In this broad-spectrum context, the names and faces of patients affected by rationing decisions are invisible among the broad choices made on behalf of groups and communities. Every once in a while, though, the media become aware of a story that they believe brings out the personal suffering of a particular patient who is deprived of a treatment allegedly because the healthcare system, in this case UK's National Health Service, cannot afford to fund it. The case of Child B is among the best known of these accounts. Her story was used to highlight the personal suffering of a single patient and her family for whom decision-makers at a health authority refused to fund an experimental treatment that might have prolonged Child B's life. The story and the judgement held by the Court of Appeal raise issues salient to the way in which rationing decisions are made.

How was the decision made?

The story of Child B illustrates that many factors are relevant to decision-making about rationing. The Court of Appeal contained four points in its judgement. These will be considered for their bearing on the general context.

Case 34 continued
The Court of Appeal's decision[9]

The Court of Appeal held:

(i) Difficult and agonizing judgements had to be made as to how the limited budget could be best allocated for the maximum advantage for the maximum number of patients. That was not a judgement for the court.
(ii) The authority had not exceeded its powers or acted unreasonably. The powers of the Court of Appeal were not such that it could substitute its own decision for that of the authority.

(iii) The decision by the hospital authority not to fund specific treatment for B on the grounds that the proposed treatment, described as experimental, would not be in her best interests and that the expenditure would not be an effective use of its limited resources, was not unlawful.
(iv) Accordingly the court could not intervene by way of judicial review.

The face of pain, or generals and particulars

The statement in section (i) undoubtedly describes the case as one of rationing of scarce resources, the resources in this case being money or the budget of the health authority in question. The judge pointed out that the decision-makers had to make 'difficult and agonizing' decisions about the economic constraints under which the health authority had to function. This is a significant point because it appeals to the natural aversion most of us feel towards applying monetary value to the lives and suffering of individuals. No doubt, the people responsible for making the decision not to fund Child B's treatment did so knowing that their decision would impact on the length of her life. In the event, doctors had given Child B only 6–8 weeks of survival, and the treatment promised a 10% chance of extending this by months. Those involved in making the decision would have had to struggle with the knowledge that they would effectively eliminate whatever small chance B had left, and shorten the time she and her family could spend together. Given our revulsion at making such determinations strictly on the basis of money, it cannot have been an easy decision.

In adjudicating a special claim on resources, by an identifiable individual, who is likely to die quite quickly if resources are not forthcoming, commissioners may feel compelled to assist, even if they would not consider the small possibility to benefit worth the cost under other circumstances, perhaps where death is not imminent.[10]

It was the identifiability of the patient in this case that brought it to media attention and which made the decision so difficult to accept. It is hard enough to cope with the knowledge that unidentifiable, nameless and faceless possible future patients will be personally affected by a decision against funding a particular treatment. However, in a situation where the patient affected is actually identifiable, has a face, a name, a family who care about her survival and an immediate need for the treatment, it will be even more difficult to say 'no'. This notion may have been what encouraged Child B's father to request the court to remove the conventional barriers that protect children from being identified in the press. His belief was that knowledge of her condition and her life would call attention to her suffering and summon enough public pressure to change the minds of the decision-makers involved. Child B was revealed as Jaymee Bowen, an articulate and endearing 10-year-old girl. It might have been a ploy of emotive manipulation, but no one can fault her father, David Bowen, for trying to do whatever was necessary to give his daughter every possible chance of extended survival. He turned the debate into a tug of war between a father's love and a utilitarian health agenda or, to put it another way, the good of the few against the good of the many. In a sense his ploy worked. After the health authority's decision was upheld in the Court of Appeal, a private benefactor donated the funds needed to permit the experimental treatment to go ahead. The results were that Jaymee Bowen lived a further few months, or as one author put it:

> This treatment enabled Jaymee to enjoy a few extra months of life. David Bowen believed that this vindicated the actions

he had taken, even though Jaymee became ill again and eventually died in May 1996.[11]

Many decisions in the healthcare context are based on general clinical judgements designed to act as guidelines or guidance for broad populations. These judgements are made on the basis of well-researched information about the adequacy of the treatment under consideration. General assertions are then formulated on the basis of the research. However, they will necessarily incorporate matters of judgement, when the facts of science are interpreted by human observers who must apply bias or prejudicial judgements to the way in which they understand what they see, or do not see, as the case may be. Think of the way an optimist sees a glass as half full while a pessimist sees the same glass as half empty. So scientists will judge what they see according to their own world-views (see Chapter 1).

This is no less true of policy and guideline decisions about healthcare. Observed facts about adequacies of treatments are coupled with judgements about their value for general populations, usually after cost–benefit analysis. The result of the generalities is that the lives of particular individuals, which are rich and complex, do not necessarily comply with the parameters assumed for populations or communities. Every patient is unique and their uniqueness will confound attempts to fit them into general contexts. The implications of this are that the individual cannot be made to fit the parameters established by the necessarily broad generalizations asserted in policy and guideline statements. Decisions such as those made about non-funding of certain treatments are challenged by individuals who can make strong claims of need such as the one made on behalf of Jaymee Bowen, who may have valued a few more weeks with her family as much as most people value many years of life.

So how can policy-makers and implementers justify their decisions affecting individual lives? Before proceeding further, consider this reflective exercise.

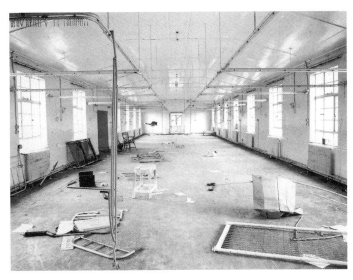

Figure 9.1
Derelict hospital, Cliveden, Berkshire – Empty Ward by Jim Harold 1992.

Offer at least two reasons the health authority might have used to justify its decision in Jaymee Bowen's case.

1.

2.

Maximizing the good

There are relevant considerations that would have made the decision not to fund the treatment somewhat easier to make. The first of these is also asserted in section (i), which points out that the decision was made for what are demonstrably utilitarian reasons. Utilitarianism advocates the greatest good for the greatest number of people (see Chapter 1, p. 4). The health authority was responsible not just for the healthcare needs of Child B, but also for meeting the healthcare needs of the entire community. The judgement accepts that the decision in Child B's case was determined on this basis and states in section (iii) that such a justification is not unlawful. Note that this does not endorse the decision, but merely states that the authority was acting within legal limitations in doing so. The health authority advocated a utilitarian moral justification for its decision. Its justification was that refusing to fund expensive treatment in this case maximized the good of a greater number of people by making the funds available to treat other cases, treatment that might be life saving and at the very least maintain or enhance quality of life. To put it more simply, the savings made by withholding funding for Jaymee Bowen's treatment were used to provide valuable healthcare to many other people.

Deontologists would have some reservations about embracing the utilitarian justification for this reason. Proponents of this duty-based moral theory would argue that maximization of good is insufficient to dismiss concerns that a child's life was devalued in favour of cost-cutting measures. Other factors need to be considered before the decision can meet deontological approval, and other factors were indeed considered. A cost–benefit analysis was performed by the health authority and presented to the Court of Appeal. Its decision was also made on the basis of the results of this analysis. It incorporated into the decision the potential good the treatment could provide the specific patient, the likelihood of this good being brought about and the potential harm the treatment could do to the patient. This brought clinical judgement into the decision process. The comparison was made between potential benefits and the foreseen harms and risks entailed by the procedure, leading to the decision that more harm than good was likely to befall the patient if the treatment was permitted to proceed. Child B would have to undergo the prolonged suffering entailed in chemotherapy, which could not be justified by the diminished chances of success. Even if it were successful, the chemotherapy would have been followed by a painful bone marrow transplant and a prolonged recovery that meant she might never enjoy a life of anything more than very low quality again before she died. None of this could be justified in accordance with duties of beneficence and non-maleficence assumed by healthcare providers. Hence the court held that it was not in Child B's interest to proceed. The ruling said:

(iii) The decision by the hospital authority not to fund specific treatment for B on the grounds that the proposed treatment, described as experimental, would not be in her best interests and that the expenditure would not be an effective use of its limited resources, was not unlawful.

The first part of the argument is clearly justifiable on deontological grounds based on a duty of care owed to the patient, or beneficence and non-maleficence. The notion that the treatment would not be in her best interests is supported by the notorious suffering and distress associated with

chemotherapy, as well as the unlikelihood of success. If the probabilities of success had been greater than 10% then the costs associated with the treatment would have been mitigated by the benefit she would have received in prolonging her life. But this was not to be the case. Thus it looked as if the doctors were acting well within their duties towards the patient to help her avoid any unnecessary suffering or burdensome treatment (see p. 96). In addition, the experimental nature of the treatment raised further ethical and clinical drawbacks. First of all, children are usually prohibited from participating in research except where the treatment will benefit them and where it is unsuitable to experiment on adults (Chapter 7, p. 130). Second, even if Jaymee Bowen had been of an age to consent to the experiment, the misery it would have inflicted would have been unlikely to justify the prolongation of her suffering.

So, from a deontological position, many duties can be called into play to justify the decision made by the health authority against funding aggressive treatment for Jaymee Bowen. The first is found in the cost–benefit analysis. Even though it is not a generally recognized tenet of deontology to accept cost–benefit analyses, which are inherently based on consequential arguments about the outcomes of expenditures, a deontologist will not reject the fundamental concern behind the principle of utility, namely to make the best use of scarce resources. This is a rationalizing principle as we have said, and as such can be viewed as an appropriate duty for a deontologist. It sets a requirement or duty not to be wasteful by inappropriately exploiting resources. Cost–benefit analyses are a means of measuring the likely success of a treatment in harmony with concerns about reasonable expenditure based on budgetary constraints. As such they offer significant information about the best use of resources, and a deontologist can appreciate this.

The second relevant duty is the one associated with the use of children in research (see Chapter 7, p. 130–133). Again, we must stay within the remit of this chapter and focus on the rationing agenda. Nevertheless, there are significant justifications for a deontological perspective on this protective regulation. A utilitarian justification for using human subjects in research trials stems from the 'maximization of good' principle underpinning utilitarianism. This theoretical position would endorse the use and even abuse of a limited number of research subjects to promote the good of other and future sufferers of the condition in question. The only way to protect the subjects is to place unconditional restraints upon researchers preventing them from performing certain types of exploitation that the community would perceive as unjustifiable. Exploitation of persons who are unable to give voluntary informed consent would be among the unjustifiable actions; therefore, to protect against this, researchers are expected to avoid enlisting incompetent subjects as far as possible, and this includes children. It is only permissible to enlist children as research subjects when: (i) it is in the child's best interest to do so because the treatment will benefit him or her personally; and (ii) when no research subject can be found among competent adults. In Jaymee Bowen's situation, the second condition was satisfied because she suffered from a condition known only to children and therefore no adult would be found to undergo the same experimental treatment. The first condition was what became the focus of the concern of all players. If the treatment could possibly be of benefit to Jaymee Bowen, then the health authority might not have been able to escape deontological accusations that the decision against funding the treatment displaced the sanctity of her life in favour of the comfort and lives of other non-identifiable potential patients. How could this be justified?

Your money or my life

Despite the results of the cost–benefit analysis, the decision not to treat still faces one final criticism from the deontologists. This criticism is founded on the simple idea that life, no matter how low its quality, is valuable in its own right. In other words, there is an inherent sanctity of life (see Chapter 6, p. 115–116). The health authority's decision not to fund the experimental treatment was founded on the expressed principle that quality of life is relevant to treatment and budgeting decisions. When David Bowen approached the health authority for funding he might not even have been considering the possibility of a cure any longer. Rather, his intention might have only been to prolong his daughter's life for as long as possible, not to prolong her suffering, but to give Jaymee and her family more time together. The health authority's decision indicates that, on balance, the diminished quality and expected length of Jaymee's life, coupled with the added hardship of further treatment, made this objectionable. The authority was left with a tragic choice, that is a choice with no possible good outcome. Either it could treat Jaymee and cause her to suffer further, or it could refuse to treat and let her die.

In this case, the idea of quality of life was considered more valid than sanctity, which creates ethical problems in its own right but can nevertheless be justified through arguments (see Chapter 6 for a discussion of these issues). For the purposes of this chapter, we will consider only whether judgements of this sort are relevant to budgetary decisions in the healthcare context. Is it legitimate to include quality of life judgements in rationing decisions or is this effectively the same thing as putting a price on life?

Quality-Adjusted Life-Years (QALYs)[12]

One famous attempt at basing resource allocation on quality of life assessments was devised for the UK in the late 1970s. The system is called QALYs, which stands for quality-adjusted life-years. QALYs were introduced in Chapter 6 in conjunction with notions of quality and quantity of life. The intention behind this approach is to place a measurable value on the quality and quantity of life. To make it possible to compare health states between individual people, their relative quality of life is determined based on an assessment of quality of health, life expectancy and the estimated cost of maintaining or improving health. One year of good health is valued as being worth 1 QALY, while death is worth 0 QALYs. Health states in between can be worth anything on the scale between 0 and 1, with the possibility of relative health states being valued at less than 0, in other words as worse than death.[13]

QALYs are mainly useful in determining the comparative value of treatments based upon their cost effectiveness. When applied in this way, the QALY can be used to measure the cost effectiveness of one form of treatment over another on the basis that one is, in practical terms, better able to produce positive effects for patients. So, if a certain illness produces a diminished health state of 0.7 QALYs and the patient is expected to live for 3 years, then the value of the quality of their lives is determined to be $0.7 \times 3 = 2.1$ QALYs. The application would then be as follows. If a treatment x can extend a life by a further 3 years and improve quality of life by 0.1, then the value of that treatment is given $0.1 \times 3 = 0.3$. If another treatment y is able to improve quality of life by 0.3 and extend survival rate by 2 years then the value of that treatment is 0.6. These numbers are not terribly useful on their own but they can be used as a crude comparison between treatment x and treatment y. On this basis, a decision can be made regarding which treatment to make readily available – namely the most effective one based on the average number of QALYs it can produce.

As a result, QALYs are most useful when attempting to compare relative health states

and the relative value of treatments that have nothing to do with one another. For instance, comparisons between treatment for neonatal heart abnormalities and continuing treatment for rheumatoid arthritis is a little like comparing apples with oranges. There are some similarities but not enough to make sense of any obvious comparison. In the former case, treatment is likely to be life saving, expensive but contained to a fixed period of time, and applied to patients in an age group who are otherwise expected to have many years of life ahead of them. In the latter, treatment is expected to be less costly but involve ongoing symptom control instead of being curative, and to affect patients in advanced years. Calculating QALYs can help make sense of the comparison because it can estimate the relative value of each of these treatments as a numerical value and permit a comparison between them. So, if one of the treatments yields 0.3 on the QALY scale while the other yields 0.6, it is clear that there is greater cost effectiveness in the one over the other.

This is where the chief problem associated with QALYs comes to light. The problem with using quality of life assessments as criteria for rationing decisions is that they are judgement based and value laden. The QALY reliance on an estimation of the quality of life experienced by different people in different states of health is therefore problematic. An accurate comparison between what people perceive to be their health state will be difficult if not impossible to determine with any accuracy. Every individual has a different perception of the good life or a good state of health. A person who has never been sick might feel devastated by a mere cold, even though most of us might think a cold is uncomfortable but does not diminish life in a significant way. People who have coped with a major disability all their lives might still judge their quality of life as good, although an outsider might perceive it to be very low. An attempt to apply numerical value to this is determined by one's perceptions at the time, hence the value one would apply to a certain health state would vary between people. So, despite the appearance of precision in this seemingly mathematical system, value judgements still interfere with its application.

Beyond this very important drawback to QALYs, David Hunter also outlined some equally important problems with QALYs in a paper published in 1993:[14,15]

- The technical base upon which QALYs have been formed is inadequate and potentially flawed
- The variability of valuations across different individuals gives rise to problems of aggregating results
- QALYs are inherently ageist, with greater values being attached to younger people
- There is a problem over the meaning of information and the approach is unable to capture the dynamic and changing nature of people's views about their health state
- The approach equates need with ability to benefit and greater importance to duration of life (life years) than to life itself
- QALYs do not distinguish between treatments that are life-enhancing (like hip replacements) and those that are life-saving (like renal replacements) and there is an attempt to equate them in some way
- QALYs potentially impact on the civil rights of individuals in terms of access to healthcare.

Hunter rightly mentions that ageism is inherent in the QALY system but should also have added that it extends to discrimination on the basis of social deprivation as well. It is an ageist system in part because it uses quantity of life as one element of the equation about value. This also raises the potential for QALYs to eliminate access to healthcare for those who are of advanced age. The older one is, the fewer number of years one can be expected to benefit from a treatment, therefore the lower the estimated value in QALYs. The calculation does not account for the chances of accident or injury shortening the life of the one that might benefit from the treatment no matter what their age. More significantly, however, the older one grows the more likely one is to have a diminished capacity to acquire a full 1 on the QALY score due to changes in health state. The natural deterioration everyone experiences from age 20 or so on potentially affects the place at which one's quality of life would score in a comparative state. QALYs turn the focus to the number of years an individual has left and the quality of life experienced during that time. The counterclaim to this is found in sanctity of life arguments, already discussed in Chapter 6, that consider life precious no matter what the quality or potential length. Whether right or wrong, this cannot be accounted for by QALYs.

Beyond age, other significant factors cause further diminishment of one's quality of life and have been demonstrated to adversely affect health. Mostly, these are socioeconomic factors, which can take the form of heightened stress levels due to struggles to meet the costs of living, depression related to abuse and deprivation, even poor access to good health services can affect an individual's quality of life and health. These are known as the comorbidity factors that impact on health and quality of life. They are often the unrecognized underlying causes of or contributors to ill health and diminished quality of life. Or, if they *are* recognized, they are frequently neglected by health services because they are considered beyond the scope of healthcare abilities, knowledge and budgets. Once again, we find no room to account for such factors in QALYs, which leads to a discrimination against those affected by comorbidity factors. These are elements that contribute to defining one's quality and even quantity of life, over which an individual might have little or no control or where social obstruction is responsible for holding them back. QALYs in effect further abuse the victims of adverse socioeconomic realities by not acknowledging their impact on quality and quantity of life and health.[16]

Proof of this was seen in 1999 league tables of healthcare in the UK.[17] Cities affected by higher amounts of social and economic deprivation also ranked very low on the healthcare league tables. This is sometimes referred to as the *inverse care law*,[18] where better care seems to gravitate toward more affluent populations whereas people living in poorer cities and neighbourhoods are further deprived by lower standards of healthcare. This form of postcode rationing cannot be supported by systems of justice that seek to alleviate the burdens of poverty and equalize distribution in a more democratic way. Yet it is perpetuated for a multitude of reasons too complex for the scope of this book. What it helps to determine is that quality of life criteria cannot be trusted to be objective enough to avoid prejudice in decision making and, as such, are too unreliable to be considered in isolation.

Implicit rationing

A significant conclusion that can be drawn from the league tables is that to some extent rationing occurs implicitly on the basis of geography and other less relevant considerations. The term 'postcode rationing' describes how some people will receive better healthcare than others simply because they live closer to well-funded hospitals, or even merely because they live in desirable neighbourhoods where doctors and other healthcare professionals choose to work. Implicit rationing occurs for a wide variety of reasons but is difficult to justify because it results in individuals being deprived without their knowledge, and hence with no means of appealing against injustice. Ideally, healthcare rationing will be explicit and an appeals process available so that anyone can know why they are being refused care and challenge the decision when they believe it to be unjust.

Was the Child B case a true case of rationing?

One final consideration ought to be made about the Child B case before we move on. In the end, is it possible that the challenge it presented was not even about rationing? One perspective that can be taken of the case reveals it as less one of rationing and more of clinical judgement.

In sections (ii) and (iii) of the Court of Appeal's decision (see p. 159), the judgement indicates that the health authority had acted reasonably within its powers, namely clinical powers to act on health-related issues. Moreover, the treatment was clinically determined to be uncertain to work and unnecessarily burdensome to the patient. Under these circumstances, it is reasonable to portray the health authority's decision as a clinical rather than economic decision based on the needs and potential benefit to the patient and not on the costs of care. If this is accurate, then it is likely that an appeals procedure could have assisted the family before it became necessary to take the case to court. That way, the Bowen family could have requested that the health authority reconsider its decision on clinical grounds and would have had recourse to presenting opposing evidence on their behalf. The outcome might not have been any different but at least it would have been argued on more appropriate grounds. In the end, if the treatment was determined to be futile, it would not have been given. Also, an appeal on clinical grounds internally before the authority would have avoided the judicial concern against overriding the decision-making power of health authorities in general.

Lessons from the Child B case

No prescribed systematic priority-setting models have been defined, which is problematic because, as a result, we end up with rationing by default. In light of this, the case of Child B raises important dimensions to the rationing debate. They include:

- Should we prefer:
  - treatment of disease versus enhancement of quality? In other words, should we prioritize cure over management?
  - proven treatments versus experimental treatments?
- The importance of distinguishing between futile and useful treatment.
- The demonstration that decisions can be clinical as well as economic.

We have discussed the case of Child B at length, and have neither exhausted the issues directly related to it nor those related to rationing in general. It will be helpful here to turn instead to a different case of rationing to help illustrate further ethical challenges and some recommendations as well.

Case 35
New flu drug

In 1999, the UK National Institute for Clinical Excellence (NICE) ruled against general prescribing of the novel influenza drug zanamivir (Relenza). The institute believed that the then current evidence from clinical trials by the manufacturer, GlaxoWellcome, suggested only a moderate benefit from the drug to otherwise healthy individuals. The drug reduces flu symptoms by about one day, and the costs of achieving this benefit are uncertain. In the absence of clear evidence of its effectiveness in high-risk patients, NICE decided against recommending general prescribing of the new drug. Rather, it pointed out that rates of flu vaccine uptake remain low, and a Department of Health spokesperson commented 'We need to do better on uptake of vaccination in people most at risk'.

But Dr John Chisholm, chairman of the BMA's General Practitioners Committee, expressed serious concerns about the implementation of the ruling. 'NICE's decision should have been given legislative force,' he said. 'The Secretary of State's failure to blacklist

the drug has done nothing to protect GPs from a potentially colossal demand for Relenza. GPs have been left between a rock and a hard place. Relenza is still available on NHS prescription, and even if GPs follow NICE's advice, as I hope they will, the prospect remains of enormous patient demand.'[19]

Professor Sir Michael Rawlins, chairman of NICE, has admitted that its decisions are 'questions of judgment, difficult to defend, difficult to teach'. Commenting specifically on NICE's rejection of zanamivir on grounds of cost, he said 'It wasn't the cost in terms of pounds, shillings, and pence, it was the cost in terms of demands on primary care.'[20]

This case helps to illustrate the salience of a stringent and open model for decision-making about rationing:

> Dr Robin Fox, editor of the *Journal of the Royal Society of Medicine*, argued that there is a lack of transparency in considering such opportunity costs. He asked 'How is the money saved by not recommending Relenza going to be spent? How do we know that it will not be used to buy another bomb?'[21]

These concerns are not unusual. They are on the minds of everyone who feels they could be a victim of a healthcare system that does not take into consideration their needs as individuals. This brings us to the central issue of justice.

Distributive justice

At the heart of resource allocation discussions is the principle of justice. Distributive justice, as distinct from criminal or civil justice, informs rationing decision theory and distribution of resources. No one has yet succeeded in issuing a comprehensive description of the concept of justice that is able to satisfy everyone. Nevertheless, it is the principle that underpins all struggles to make morally acceptable rationing decisions and the disagreement is evident from our failure to develop any single satisfactory system.

The principles of medical ethics described in Chapter 1 help to reveal the inherent conflicts involved in rationing and distributive justice. To review, the principles involved in resource distribution and allocation issues are:

- Utility:
  - resources are (necessarily) finite
  - make the best use of resources
- Justice:
  - distributional justice: how to best distribute resources
  - fairness characterized as equality of access[22]
- Autonomy:
  - respect for the individual as self-determining and self-governing
  - individual's right to make self-regarding choices
- Beneficence/non-maleficence:
  - help, do good/do no harm.

The principles in conflict over rationing reveal that autonomy and beneficence need to be balanced with justice and utility to keep the interests of the few or one in harmony with the good of the many. Applications of justice attempt to harmonize the good of the few with the good of the many. Distributive justice asserts a need for fairness in allocation of resources. But what does fairness mean? There is a degree of consensus among philosophers and health economists that justice as fairness must extend beyond clear-cut equality of distribution. Equal distribution would mean the parsing out of health resources in exactly the same quantities to each person regardless of need, eligibility or capacity to benefit. While this is morally sound in certain contexts, it is demonstrably inappropriate in the healthcare context.

Where all people have an equal potential to benefit from a resource it makes sense to disperse that resource equally, otherwise some people will lose out for unjustifiable reasons. This is usually described as discrimination. For example, all humans have an equal need for clean water. It is therefore morally unjustifiable to prevent some people from having access to clean water while making it accessible to others. Equal distribution is therefore the most ethically justifiable means of allocating clean water in a community, as this is the only way to prevent discrimination.

The same is not true of healthcare resources. Not everyone can benefit from healthcare resources to the same extent as others. For example, people in good health will not benefit to the same extent from use of healthcare resources as those with acute or long-term illness. As a result, it would be a waste of resources to distribute the same amount to those who will not need them as to those who need them to preserve their quality of life or even to keep them alive at all. A more suitable method of distribution is to ensure that resources are delivered to those who will benefit from them in some way (even if it does not save their lives). This means directing health resources towards those who need them, and withholding resources from those who will not need them. This does not involve strong discrimination, as healthy people will not usually make claims for use of resources they do not need or want.

Needs, wants and access

There is a sense in which equality is relevant in healthcare, though, and this is in the ability to access healthcare resources when required. There can exist a morally justifiable system that makes it possible to access healthcare resources when needed but which does not distribute these equally. Each according to his or her need is the best way to characterize this style of distributive justice, with the understanding that everyone still has an equal opportunity to access healthcare resources when they do require them.

Although this appears to be a simple and self-evident method of solving problems of distributive justice, it suffers from one significant flaw. Namely, there is no clear means of judging with certainty the difference between a legitimate need and a desire, preference or want. Once again we are faced with the problem of value judgements interfering with resource decisions. Needs are important but one person's need is another person's luxury, and this occurs in a variety of positions on the scale between need and desire.

> List three things you believe everyone needs:
>
> 1.
> 2.
> 3.
>
> List three things you believe people desire but do not need:
>
> 1.
> 2.
> 3.
>
> List three things that you believe are ambiguous needs or desires:
>
> 1.
> 2.
> 3.

The difference between needs and desires is surprisingly difficult to determine. Some things are relatively straightforward, such as the need for clean air or clean water. Needs are frequently associated with rights for this reason because they are identified as the basic requirements for existence: things to which everyone can claim to have a right. However, the clarity of distinction between needs and desires blurs as we try to list what the basic needs are. In some cultures, the need for a certain amount of education is a basic requirement for healthy functioning in

society. For others, the freedom to farm land or to travel as nomadic cultures do is of equal importance. Individuals claim rights to such basic needs, which confers duties upon others to provide or at least not prevent their access. However, one reason rights disputes occur is precisely because there is disagreement about the identification of needs. Some countries assert the basic right to healthcare, others deny that healthcare is a right. Systems of the first sort usually make medical care available without fees, preferring to place the burden of payment on society as a whole rather than on individuals who might not have the means to pay for care. Nationalized health systems like those in the UK and Canada are examples of such systems. Aneurin Bevan, Labour Minister of Health and the leading architect of the NHS, based his proposal for socialized medicine on the reasoning illustrated by the following quote:

> Illness is neither an indulgence for which people have to pay nor an offence for which they should be punished but a misfortune, the cost of which should be shared by the community.[23]

Other countries have preferred to consider healthcare not to be a right. Countries such as the US require individuals to pay for their health care, either through private insurance or on their own. Only when a person can no longer afford to pay for care does the state provide any assistance. In other countries, no state assistance is provided. Justifications for these systems usually hinge on arguments indicating the failures of socialized models of medical care. They point to overly long waiting lists and restricted availability or quality of care in tax-based healthcare systems. Arguments in favour or against either style are beyond the scope of this text. The point is raised simply to illustrate the difficulty in determining the difference between needs and wants with clarity, as here again we are faced with the uncertainty of value-based judgements. Distinguishing what is a need from a want is value based and therefore no less uncertain than other issues already discussed in this chapter.

One thing emerges from the analysis, and that is that for a system to be just, the burden of deprivation ought to be distributed equally. This way, if some needs will not be met then the burden will not fall on just a few members of the population.

Ability to benefit or need

If value-based decisions such as needs or quality of life are too uncertain for rationing decisions, then what more appropriate criteria can be relied upon? One classic proposal is decision on the basis of ability to benefit. By this argument, resources will be given only to patients who are likely to improve from treatment. The justification is founded on the notion that it makes sense to use resources only where they will be of benefit. This is countered by arguments that suggest healthcare resources are best distributed according to need, but this, we have seen, is problematic because it is difficult to distinguish between needs and wants. Which of these criteria is more appropriate to consider in the context of healthcare? Not surprisingly, each has its benefits and drawbacks.[24]

If we base rationing decisions on the ability of the patient to improve with the treatment then, on the up-side, we will have a great deal of funding for proven effective treatments for curable diseases, because they constitute the best value for money. Thus, priority will be given to patients who are most able to benefit from treatment, and this will usually mean directing funds at curable illness. The problem with this is that it places patients with a lesser ability to benefit from treatment very low on the prioritizing list. In other words, patients dying from incurable diseases and those suffering from long-term incurable illness will be less likely to receive care due to economic shortages because they

are less likely to benefit from care. So, for example, patients with AIDS who required expensive treatment for, say, glaucoma, will be less likely to receive the treatment because their life expectancy is so short. But there will be plenty of money to spend on antibiotics for streptococcal infections in otherwise healthy individuals because it is such an effective treatment. Resources for research will be debatable under this theory, although there would be pressure to prove the effectiveness of treatment because this will determine whether or not they will be used. On the other hand, preference will be given to treatments already proven to work, so funding for development could become scarce.

Conversely, we could base rationing decisions on need. This would mean responding to those who are most unwell, treating patients regardless of ability to improve or be cured. In a recent paper,[25] John Harris defended the idea that public health systems ought to respond to patient needs regardless of their ability to benefit from the treatment or the length of life they can expect as a result of the treatment. This is a defiant position to embrace. Indeed, Harris was writing in response to arguments that suggest his position leads to false conclusions.[26] Harris states that the traditional arguments in favour of considering the ability to benefit from a treatment are fundamentally immoral. He says:

The principle that each individual is entitled to an equal opportunity to benefit from any public healthcare system, and that this entitlement is proportionate neither to the size of their chance of benefiting, nor to the quality of the benefit, nor to the length of lifetime remaining in which that benefit may be enjoyed, runs counter to most current thinking about the allocation of resources for healthcare. It is my contention that any system of prioritisation of the resources available for healthcare or for rationing such resources must be governed by this principle.[27]

The advantage to this is that illness and diseases such as AIDS, multiple sclerosis, Huntington's disease and spina bifida would be treated despite the patient's poor prognosis or incurability. However, it would also cause us to treat those most in need and perhaps leave few resources for less apparently significant illnesses such as colds or a bad knee. Moreover, the patients who did receive the resources would not necessarily benefit from the treatment for long periods of time, and some might even die before the benefits had been felt. We would also be deterred from preventive interventions because they do not reveal themselves as urgent needs in the same way that acute illnesses do. Thus measures such as vaccination programmes and community interventions about poor housing or unclean water, which are the cause of so much illness, would be placed in low priority compared with acute illnesses such as heart disease.

A compromise is possible, which ensures some acute needs are responded to while less acute illness is not ignored. But this too has its drawbacks. It is desirable to treat at all ends of the spectrum of need, regardless of ability to improve or benefit, otherwise we fail to try where little hope exists, or fail to treat where the benefit is comparatively small but still greatly appreciated by the patient. Palliative medicine is an excellent example of care that can appear less beneficial because it does not aim to cure. It is clear that people in need of palliative care are in need of treatment but equally clear that many will not be cured with it. How could we refuse this treatment? Perhaps we should not. Perhaps treating even in these circumstances can be justifiable because it promotes more caring attitudes than those formed by theories that would prioritize treatment only where it can cure successfully. This can then be balanced

by recognition of when it is futile to impose treatment and therefore allocate resources more rationally by using them only where they are truly necessary. It also recognizes that the ability to benefit can be contingent on one's perspective. We measure success in different ways. In the case of Child B, the idea of prolonging whatever precious time could be made available to Jaymee and her family meant the benefit was measured in days or hours rather than months or years, but was still highly valued. This indicates the potential drawback to the compromise approach, because it doesn't really solve the problem of how we ought to prioritize when resources are scarce.

Desert

Prioritizing in resource allocation can be made on the basis of desert or merit, but such an approach is deeply flawed. Decisions based on desert would be a means of deciding who ought to receive healthcare based on assessment of their worthiness for treatment. Thus decisions about allocation of resources would be based on the question: who deserves it most? The criteria for assessment would then rest on fairly shaky grounds. Would we provide care to all who pay for it, either directly or via taxes or insurance policies? Or do we provide care to those who have earned it by helping others or doing good deeds in the community or the rest of the world? Would priority be given to sick or injured heroes or to the victims they rescue? Can we give care only to people who have taken the necessary precautions not to become ill? What if they get sick anyway? What about those that self-inflict illness, for example smokers or people who engage in risky activities such as bungee jumping?

The problem comes in determining who deserves healthcare. It is no easier if we try to reformulate the question in the negative by asking who does not deserve to receive healthcare. Either way, the list of determining factors will be impossible to construct without engendering contradictions to the moral principles embraced by health carers. Primary among these is the duty of care as represented by beneficence and non-maleficence. The point of healthcare is not to judge who deserves care; the point of health-care is to care for those who are ill. Determination of desert is the remit of social and legal justice and is the realm of politicians and judges. Doctors can play a role in lobbying or informing the debate, but they must not become the judges of issues outside the realm of healthcare.

The reasons for this are manifold. First, doctors are not trained to be judges of moral character or desert. It is the doctor's duty to provide care to the best of their abilities and not to spend time deciding whether the patient deserves to benefit from the resources used to provide it or not. More importantly, however, the decision to make desert a determinant of reception of health-care would lead to conflict and injustices. For every criterion one could propose in favour of desert, a group would emerge as unjustly treated by the ensuing deprivation. Consider the following examples.

Ability to pay
If we include only those who can pay, or have contributed to taxes, then we exclude those who are unable to pay, such as children. We could adjust this by providing care also for those with a potential to pay, but this would exclude patients who will never be able to pay, e.g. terminally ill children like Child B, or people with severe disabilities. In such circumstances it conflicts with the notion of a just and beneficent society to refuse help simply because the patient cannot contribute and never will, although they have legitimate healthcare needs.

Exclude risk takers
If we limit resource expenditures to those who do not engage in risk-taking activities we face a problem of delineation: namely that, in practice, it will be difficult to draw a line between risky and safe behaviour. If riding a motorcycle without a helmet is risky then what about skiing or skydiving? Is crossing the street or driving a car considered risky behaviour? Even though most people do these things, they are notoriously very dangerous, as the chances of being killed or injured by a car or on the street are very high. Even taking the bus to work in the morning increases your risk of catching a cold from the stranger standing next to you. Where will we draw the line? This is a real challenge because we hesitate to prevent people from taking all risks as it too greatly confines their freedom of choice and autonomous rights to live (and die) in the way they choose or the way that most suits their values and ambitions. A preference for liberty and freedom of choice will inhibit, although not eliminate, social intervention of risk-taking behaviour. Some social intervention does exist in the form of laws that are paternalistic in nature. Helmet and safety belt laws are two examples of such. These laws interfere with individuals' rights to free choice on the ground that doing so is in the best interests of those individuals affected. However, even paternalistic laws can be shown to stem from social requirements of the principle of utility because everyone benefits if severe accidents are prevented and the health resources are not drained as a result. If this is the justification for the law then it is not, strictly speaking, paternalistic because the restriction is aimed at benefiting the community of health resource users, not the individuals themselves. But this brings us back to individual liberties and one's freedom to do as one wishes.

Self-inflicted illness[28]
People who smoke are frequently listed as undeserving users of health resources because smoking is clearly a risky behaviour. The illnesses associated with smoking are sometimes considered to be self-inflicted because they can be prevented by abstaining

from or limiting intake of tobacco, and this information is widely known. Yet people persist in smoking and questions about whether smokers deserve treatment have been seriously considered as part of a rationing agenda. But this conclusion feels distinctly unjust. Many of us knowingly use unhealthy products and foods despite understanding how seriously they can affect our health over time. Should we all be blamed for the ill-health that befalls us as a result? Doing so would be virtually impossible. To begin with, it would be impossible to gauge how all foods and household products affect us. Most foods have been discovered to have carcinogenic or otherwise unhealthy properties at one time or another, and new information emerges about this every day. It is difficult to know to what degree we can be said to be responsible for our exposure to and intake of dangerous substances, and even more difficult to determine how each of us will be affected by exposure given our unique genetic make-up. Moreover, many people claim to be addicted to unhealthy things such as cigarettes and as such are victims of their ill-health rather than perpetrators.

We all manufacture our own poor health to some degree, but it is our right to do so, as these are our own bodies. Ideally, we will treat them as well as possible but, failing that, at least we are free to treat them any way we choose. This is autonomy in its simplest and purest sense, autonomy over one's own body and the freedom we recognize as a right to do as we want.

These arguments demonstrate that desert is a seriously flawed method of making rationing decisions. No best system has been defined.

Who should decide?

Alongside the question of how decisions ought to be made come considerations of who ought to make decisions about

rationing. Doctors are sometimes described as the gatekeepers of medical resources, determining, presumably on the basis of clinical judgement, what share of the health resources each patient will receive. When patients consult their GP, one of three outcomes usually arises: (i) they are given a prescription; (ii) they are referred to a specialist; or (iii) they are not given any active treatment at all. Any one of these has a bearing on the resource budget, but that is not likely to be the intention behind the conclusion. More than likely, the decision is made based on the doctor's determination of what is best for the patient, preferably after discussion with that patient and seeking informed consent. It would be worrying to patients to believe that their doctor might be basing decisions not on the patient's best interests but with a view to the best interests of society instead. The principle of utility urges healthcare practitioners to do just that: to consider the interests of society by making best use of resources. In essence, utility pits the good of the individual against the good of the community. If doctors are expected to maintain this balance then they will sometimes have to sacrifice the best interests of the patient before them to protect the interests of abstract members of the community. This feels intuitively wrong. Sometimes the individual needs someone to advocate on their behalf to ensure they receive what they need and deserve. In the healthcare context it is the healthcare professional who might be best suited to do this.

This is not to say that doctors should not participate in rationing decisions. It only means that bedside rationing by individual doctors regarding particular patients ought to be eliminated. Instead, rationing decisions and resource allocation are better made by groups of individuals whose remit is to consider the interests of entire communities while also recognizing the interests of the few who might need special consideration. Groups such as the Rationing Agenda Group in the UK make decisions that inform public policy about the best use of resources and determine the most acceptable means of making rationing decisions. The groups are usually multidisciplinary, involving doctors, nurses, managers, economists, politicians, lawyers, philosophers, clergy and patients.

No matter who is included, it is essential that policies are transparent and justifiable. Decision makers must develop and reveal the reasons for their decisions and must be able to respond to individual needs.

The Oregon Health Plan

This degree of openness and accountability suggests another possibility for rationing policy. This is to take a democratic approach to determining which conditions will receive treatment. Such an attempt has been made in the American state of Oregon. The Oregon Health Plan[29] was the first public process of priority setting in healthcare. The Oregon authorities used both expert and democratic means of creating a list of state-fundable medical conditions. Their criteria were based initially on the feasibility of treatments informed by cost–benefit analysis. This generated a list of treatments considered worthy of state support. The list was then distributed for consideration to all members of the Oregon electorate, regardless of health or other status. Citizens were asked to prioritize conditions they considered to be worthy of state-supported healthcare.

The experiment was to a large degree successful and has been used in modified form since. However, it does have some drawbacks. Most significantly, the Oregon list includes cancer and heart disease but ignores rare or stigmatized diseases.[30]

International issues: the global picture

For one-third of the world the question of scarce healthcare resources focuses on high and new technological advances, such as organ transplantation, MRI and CAT scans, and genetic research. In the other two-thirds of the world the resources being rationed include fresh water supplies and low-tech interventions such as vaccinations and the treatment of parasitic diseases that perpetuate famines.[31]

Priorities are different depending on the context and country the decision is to be made in. The average annual expenditure on healthcare per person have been estimated to be as follows:[32]

- the UK: $1000+
- the US: $2000+
- developing nations: $6–9.

The disparate nature of these figures is obvious and disturbing. It could be that these inequalities will never be resolved and the ability to spend on healthcare might always vary between countries. The question remains as to how much responsibility must fall to wealthier nations to assist financially and health-deprived nations.

An element of goodwill is required of any health professional. The desire to use skills and knowledge to come to the aid of those who need them is almost essential to the profession. But to what extent can it be required and how far must it extend? Most of us would agree that charity has intrinsic value but there is little agreement of how much and who ought to benefit from it. Some theorists argue that there is no need for commitment to do good outside of one's immediate community. We certainly could not fault the doctor who comes to the aid of those who appeal directly. But is this enough? These days, there is considerable argument for saying that the world community is equally deserving of care, especially when we now have clear images via the media of the suffering experienced in the so-called developing nations or the urgent appeals from victims of natural disaster.

In a paper published in the 1970s, the controversial philosopher Peter Singer suggested that a little bit was simply not enough because knowledge of the suffering of others placed a moral obligation upon us to respond until the suffering is over. He begins his famous paper *Famine, affluence and morality*[33] with 'As I write this, in November 1971, people are dying in East Bengal from lack of food, shelter, and medical care.' As he continues, the lines between duty and charity begin to blur and one is left with the conclusion that we must give all we can to assist. We must give up any luxuries and realign our priorities to come to the aid of those who need it, regardless of their nearness or distance. As resources are finite and more immediate, less urgent, responsibilities urge us to respond, it might be easier to contain the number of those who can be said to have a moral claim over particular sets of resources. Singer disagrees and ultimately states:

> If it is within our power to prevent something very bad from happening, without thereby sacrificing anything else morally significant, we ought, morally, to do it.

Singer's position has been criticized for two reasons. First, critics argue that charity must be kept distinct from duty to retain its intrinsically valuable characteristic. This is because charitable acts are considered to contribute to the improvement of a society by their very existence. So removing the possibility of acting charitably by turning such acts into duties would diminish the worth of our social interactions. Duties are expected and people can be blamed for not performing them, but we do not expect praise for their performance. However, charitable acts are praiseworthy because they go beyond the scope of one's expected duties.

Second, concerns arise about the degree to which we can be expected to give to other people with whom we will never have any contact. Recall the old adage that charity begins at home. We give to a certain extent

but save to assist those in our more immediate surroundings. Singer's critics argue that it is not inappropriate to give preference to those more immediate to us.

There is no clear way of knowing to what degree our responsibilities are owed to others and how much charity is enough. Organizations such as the World Medical Association (WMA), the World Health Organization (WHO), Médecins sans Frontières[34] and MEDACT[35] make it possible for health carers to extend the boundaries of the duty of care beyond the national into the international. These groups provide opportunities for healthcare professionals and students to respond to the needs of patients outside their own borders. No healthcare professional is required to participate in these initiatives but it remains to be argued whether they ought to for the sake of justice.

Conclusion: the elements of a just healthcare system

To conclude, the following are some general principles that can be considered as guidelines for morally acceptable rationing decisions:

- universal access
- access to an 'adequate level of care'
- access without excessive burdens
- fair distribution of financial costs ensuring universal access and access to an adequate level of care
- fair distribution of the burdens of rationing
- capacity for improvement toward a more just system.[36]

The same arguments have been strongly put by many who believe that, regardless of underpinning principles, no method of resource allocation can be ethically justifiable if it does not acknowledge the following general considerations:

- that there is a difference between implicit and explicit rationing
- rationing policies must be subject to accountability and transparency
- rationing judgements must be justifiable
- the decision makers must have arguments to support their decisions
- anyone should have access to information about decisions and criteria for judgements
- an appeals process should be available for patients who believe themselves to be unfairly treated by policy decisions.

Ultimately, we are left with one significant question. That is, is it acceptable to withhold or withdraw medical treatment purely for economic reasons? Our only answer seems to be that it might be necessary to do so, but we hope it will be done in a fair and just manner.

Notes and references

1 Buchanan A. Privatisation and just health care. Bioethics 1995; 9:220–239.

2 See: Hope T. The best is the enemy of the good – can research ethics learn from rationing? J Medical Ethics 2000; 26:417–418 and Hope T. QALYs, lotteries and veils: the story so far. J Medical Ethics 1996; 22:195–196.

3 Julian Tudor-Hart said: 'With NHS costs at roughly £6 a tablet and research, development and production costs estimated at around one hundredth of that (still leaving a good profit, granted wider prescription), I find it curious that any health economist can still talk as though resources were finite and beyond question.' Hoolet, Autumn 1999:12.

4 From the argument in Downie R, Calman K. Healthy respect. Oxford: Oxford University Press; 1994.

5 Alan Milburn, Labour Secretary of State for health, as quoted in Yamey G. News extra: health secretary admits that NHS rationing is government policy. Br Med J 2000; 320:10.

6 The euro has been one such attempt.

7 The Oregon Experiment in the US is a good example of this, as will be expanded upon on page 174.

8 Nelson-Jones R, Burton F. Medical negligence case law. 2nd edn. London: Butterworths; 1995:501. See also: Ham C, Pickard S. Tragic choices in health care: the case of child B. London: King's Fund; 1998

and Thornton S. Personal view: the child B case – reflections of a chief executive. Br Med J 1997; 314:1838.

9 Nelson-Jones R, Burton F. Medical negligence case law. 2nd edn. London: Butterworths; 1995:501.

10 Draper H, Tunna K. Ethics and values for commissioners. Leeds: Nuffield Institute Health; 1996:44.

11 Ham C. Tragic choices in health care: lessons from the child B case. Br Med J 1999; 319:1258–1261.

12 For good discussions on QALYs see Downie R, Macnaughton J. Clinical judgement: evidence in practice. Oxford: Oxford University Press; 2000.

13 Newport CP. So what is a QALY? Bandolier, February 1996:24–27. Available: http://www.ebando.com/band24/b24-7.html

14 Hunter D. The mysteries of health gain. In: Harrison H, ed. Health care UH 1992/93. London: King's Fund Institute; 1993:99–105.

15 Hunter D. The mysteries of health gain. In: Harrison H, ed. Health care UH 1992/93. London: King's Fund Institute; 1993:101

16 See: Macintyre S. Modernising the NHS: prevention and the reduction of health inequalities. Br Med J 2000; 320:1399–1400 and Klein P. The second phase of priority setting. Br Med J 1998; 1000–1007.

17 League tables drawn up on the basis of research performed by The King's Fund and Channel 4.

18 Tudor-Hart J. The inverse care law. Lancet 1971; i:405–412.

19 Yamey G. Dobson backed NICE ruling on flu drug. Br Med J 1999; 319:1024.

20 Yamey G. Chairman of NICE admits that its judgements are hard to defend. Br Med J 1999; 319:1222.

21 Yamey G. Chairman of NICE admits that its judgements are hard to defend. Br Med J 1999; 319:1222.

22 Daniels N. The case of private insurance. Second international conference on priorities in health care. London: 8–10 October 1998.

23 Bevan A.

24 New, L-G. Rationing in the NHS: principles and pragmatism. London: Baillière-Tindall; 1996.

25 Harris J. Justice and equal opportunities in health care. Bioethics 1999; 13(5):392–404.

26 Savulescu J. Consequentialism, reason, value and justice. Bioethics 1998; 12(3):212–235.

27 Harris J. Justice and equal opportunities in health care. Bioethics 1999; 13(5):392–404.

28 Higgs R. Human frailty should not be penalised. Br Med J 1993; 306:1049.

29 For a history of The Oregon Health Plan described by the state legislature, see: http://ohppr.das.state.or.us/pubs/ohp_summ.htm and http://ohppr.das.state.or.us/pubs/list_sum.htm

See also: Ham C. Retracing the Oregon Trail: the experience of rationing and the Oregon Health Plan. Br Med J 1998; 316:1965–1969.

30 For the complete list, see: http://ohppr.das.state.or.us/pubs/list.htm

31 See: Taylor D. Poor world health and rich world wealth. Br Med J 2001; 322:629–630 and MacDonald R. Providing clean water: lessons from Bangladesh. Br Med J 2001; 322:626–627.

32 See World Development Report 1993: investing in health. Available at: http://www.worldbank.org/wdr/previous

33 Singer P. Famine, affluence and morality. Philosophy and Public Affairs 1972; 1(3) (Spring).

34 The Médecins sans Frontières website is available at: http://www.medecinssansfrontieres.com/

35 The MEDACT website is available at: http://www.medact.org/

36 Buchanan A. Privatisation and just health care. Bioethics 1995; 9:220–239.

Appendix 1
Common ethical codes

When researching the various 'ethical codes' that have been produced we spoke to a number of doctors who practise in different countries. It became apparent that codes of ethics tend to be a product of secular societies. In countries with a generally held religious tradition, such codes are less prevalent because the way medicine is practised is governed by God's laws.

We think it is of interest to set out some of the more widely accepted codes.

The oath of a Muslim physician

Praise be to Allah [God], the Teacher, the Unique, Majesty of the Heavens, the Exalted, the Glorious, Glory be to Him, the Eternal Being Who created the Universe and all the creatures within, and the only Being Who contained the infinity and the eternity. We serve no other god besides Thee and regard idolatry as an abominable injustice.

Give us the strength to be truthful, honest, modest, merciful and objective.

Give us the fortitude to admit our mistakes, to amend our ways and to forgive the wrongs of others.

Give us the wisdom to comfort and counsel all towards peace and harmony.

Give us the understanding that ours is a profession sacred that deals with your most precious gifts of life and intellect.

Therefore, make us worthy of this favoured station with honor, dignity and piety so that we may devote our lives in serving mankind, poor or rich, literate or illiterate, Muslim or non-Muslim, black or white with patience and tolerance with virtue and reverence, with knowledge and vigilance, with Thy love in our hearts and compassion for Thy servants, Thy most precious creation.

Hereby we take this oath in Thy name, the Creator of all the Heavens and the earth and follow Thy counsel as Thou has revealed to Prophet Mohammad (Peace Be Upon Him):

'Whosoever killeth a human being, not in lieu of another human being nor because of mischief on earth, it is as if he hath killed all mankind. And if he saveth a human life, he hath saved the life of all mankind.' (The Holy Qur'an, Chapter 5, Verse 35)

This medical oath, which is a composite from the historical and contemporary writings of physicians of Islamic World, was officially adopted by Islamic Medical Association of North America in 1977.

Oath of Maimonides

The eternal providence has appointed me to watch over the life and health of Thy creatures. May the love for my art actuate me at all time; may neither avarice nor miserliness, nor thirst for glory or for a great reputation engage my mind; for the enemies of truth and philanthropy could easily decieve me and make me forgetful of my lofty aim of doing good to Thy children.

May I never see in the patient anything but a fellow creature in pain.

Grant me the strength, time and opportunity always to correct what I have aquired, always to extendits domain; for knowledge is immense and the spirit of man can extend indefintely to enrich itself daily with new requirements.

Today he can discover his errors of yesterday and tomorrow he can obtain a new light on what he thinks himself sure of today. Oh, God, Thou has appointed me to watch over the life and death of Thy creatures; here am I ready for my vocation and now I turn unto my calling.

The hippocratic oath

The old Hippocratic oath ~425BC

I swear by Apollo the physician, and Aesculapius and Health and All-heal, and all the gods and goddesses, that, according to my ability and judgment, I will keep this oath and stipulation – to reckon him who taught me this Art equally dear to me as my parents, to share my substance with him, and relieve his necessities if required; to look upon his offspring in the same footing as my own brothers, and to teach them this Art, if they shall wish to learn it, without fee or stipulation, and that by percept, lecture, and every other mode of instruction, I will impart a knowledge of the Art to my own sons, and those of my teachers, and to disciples bound by a

The new Hippocratic oath ~1998AD

I promise that my medical knowledge will be used to benefit people's health. Patients are my first concern. I will listen to them, and provide the best care I can. I will be honest, respectful, and compassionate towards patients.

I will do my best to help *anyone* in medical need, in emergencies. I will make every effort to ensure that the rights of all patients are respected, including vulnerable groups who lack means of making their needs known.

I will exercise my professional judgment as independently as possible,

Oath and law of Hippocrates

From "Harvard Classics Volume 38" Copyright 1910 by P.F. Collier and Son.

This text is placed in the Public Domain, June 1993.

INTRODUCTORY NOTE

HIPPOCRATES, the celebrated Greek physician, was a contemporary of the historian Herodotus. He was born in the island of Cos between 470 and 460 B.C., and belonged to the family that claimed descent from the mythical Aesculapius, son of Apollo. There was already along medical tradition in Greece before his day, and this he is supposed to have inherited chiefly through his predecessor Herodicus; and he enlarged his education by extensive travel. He is said, though the evidence is stipulation and oath according to the law of medicine, but to none other.

I will follow that system of regimen, which, according to my ability and judgment, I consider for the benefit of my patients, and abstain from whatever is deleterious and mischievous.

I will give no deadly medicine to anyone if asked, nor suggest any such counsel; and in like manner I will not give to a woman a pessary to produce abortion. With purity and with holiness I will pass my life and practice my Art.

I will not cut persons labouring under the stone, but will leave this to be done by men who are practitioners of this work. Into whatever houses I enter, I will go into them for the benefit of the sick, and will abstain from every voluntary act of mischief and corruption; and, further, from the seduction of females, or males, of freemen or slaves.

Whatever, in connection with my professional practice, not in connection with it, I see or hear, in the life of men, which ought not to be spoken of abroad, I will not divulge, as reckoning that all such should be kept secret.

While I continue to keep this Oath unviolated, may it be granted to me to enjoy life and the practice of the Art,

uninfluenced by political pressure or by the social standing of my patient. I will not put personal profit or advancement above my duty to my patient.

I recognize the special value of human life, but I also know that prolongation of human life is not the only aim of health care. If I agree to perform abortion,* I agree that it should take place only within an ethical and legal framework.

I will not provide treatments which are pointless or harmful, or which an informed and competent patient refuses. I will help** patients find the information and support they want to make decisions on their care.

I will answer as truthfully as I can, and respect patients' decisions, unless that puts others at risk of substantial*** harm. If I cannot agree with their requests, I will explain why.

If my patients have limited mental awareness, I will still encourage them to participate in decisions as much as they feel able. I will do my best to maintain confidentiality about all patients.

If there are overriding reasons which prevent my keeping a patient's confidentiality I will explain them. I will recognize the limits of my knowledge and seek advice from colleagues

unsatisfactory, to have taken part in the efforts to check the great plague which devastated Athens at the beginning of the Peloponnesian war. He died at Larissa between 380 and 360 BC. The works attributed to Hippocrates are the earliest extant Greek medical writings, but very many of them are certainly not his. Some five or six, however, are generally granted to be genuine, and among these is the famous 'Oath.' This interesting document shows that in his time physicians were already organized into a corporation or guild, with regulations for the training of disciples, and with an esprit de corps and a professional ideal which, with slight exceptions, can hardly yet be regarded as out of date. One saying occurring in the words of Hippocrates has achieved universal currency, though few who quote it today are aware that it originally referred to the art of the physician. It is the first of his 'Aphorisms': 'Life is short, and the Art long; the occasion fleeting; experience fallacious, and judgment difficult'. The physician must not only be prepared to do what is right himself, but also to make the patient, the attendants, and externals cooperate.

THE LAW OF HIPPOCRATES

1. Medicine is of all the arts the most noble; but, owing to the ignorance of those who practice it, and of those who, inconsiderately, form a

respected by all men, in all times. But should I trespass and violate this Oath, may the reverse be my lot.

when needed. I will acknowledge my mistakes.

I will do my best to keep myself and my colleagues informed of new developments, and ensure that poor standards or bad practices are exposed to those who can improve them.

I will show respect for all those with whom I work and be ready to share my knowledge by teaching others what I know. I will use my training and professional standing to improve the community in which I work.

I will treat patients equitably and support a fair and humane distribution of health resources. I will try to influence positively authorities whose policies harm public health.

I will oppose policies which breach internationally accepted standards of human rights. I will strive to change laws which are contrary to patients' interests or to my professional ethics.

While I continue to keep this Oath unviolated, may it be granted to me to enjoy life and the practice of the Art, respected by all, in all times.

After the BMA's *Revised Hippocratic Oath*, with changes: *The BMA draft did not cater for those believing that

judgment of them, it is at present far behind all the other arts. Their mistake appears to me to arise principally from this, that in the cities there is no punishment connected with the practice of medicine (and with it alone) except disgrace, and that does not hurt those who are familiar with it. Such persons are the figures which are introduced in tragedies, for as they have the shape, and dress, and personal appearance of an actor, but are not actors, so also physicians are many in title but very few in reality.

2. Whoever is to acquire a competent knowledge of medicine, ought to be possessed of the following advantages: a natural disposition; instruction; a favorable position for the study; early tuition; love of labour; leisure. First of all, a natural talent is required; for, when Nature leads the way to what is most excellent, instruction in the art takes place, which the student must try to appropriate to himself by reflection, becoming an early pupil in a place well adapted for instruction. He must also bring to the task a love of labour and perseverance, so that the instruction taking root may bring forth proper and abundant fruits.

3. Instruction in medicine is like the culture of the productions of the earth. For

abortion is unethical. **The BMA wording was stronger here, requiring us to *ensure* that patients actually *receive* this information (often an impossibility). ***The word *substantial* has been added to prevent a serious breach of confidentiality in the name of a slight benefit to another party. Contrary to the BMA's version, the last paragraph about enjoying life has been inserted from the old oath. Other changes are minor.

our natural disposition, is, as it were, the soil; the tenets of our teacher are, as it were, the seed; instruction in youth is like the planting of the seed in the ground at the proper season; the place where the instruction is communicated is like the food imparted to vegetables by the atmosphere; diligent study is like the cultivation of the fields; and it is time which imparts strength to all things and brings them to maturity.

4. Having brought all these requisites to the study of medicine, and having acquired a true knowledge of it, we shall thus, in travelling through the cities, be esteemed physicians not only in name but in reality. But inexperience is a bad treasure, and a bad fund to those who possess it, whether in opinion or reality, being devoid of self-reliance and contentedness, and the nurse both of timidity and audacity. For timidity betrays a want of powers, and audacity a lack of skill. They are, indeed, two things, knowledge and opinion, of which the one makes its possessor really to know, the other to be ignorant.

5. Those things which are sacred, are to be imparted only to sacred persons; and it is not lawful to impart them to the profane until they have been initiated into the mysteries of the science.

Appendix 2

The Universal Declaration of Human Rights

On 10 December 1948, the General Assembly of the United Nations adopted and proclaimed the Universal Declaration of Human Rights, the full text of which appears in the following pages. Following this historic act the Assembly called upon all Member countries 'to publicize the text of the Declaration and to cause it to be disseminated, displayed, read and expounded principally in schools and other educational institutions, without distinction based on the political status of countries or territories'.

Preamble

Whereas recognition of the inherent dignity and of the equal and inalienable rights of all members of the human family is the foundation of freedom, justice and peace in the world,

Whereas disregard and contempt for human rights have resulted in barbarous acts which have outraged the conscience of mankind, and the advent of a world in which human beings shall enjoy freedom of speech and belief and freedom from fear and want has been proclaimed as the highest aspiration of the common people,

Whereas it is essential, if man is not to be compelled to have recourse, as a last resort, to rebellion against tyranny and oppression, that human rights should be protected by the rule of law,

Whereas it is essential to promote the development of friendly relations between nations,

Whereas the peoples of the United Nations have in the Charter reaffirmed their faith in fundamental human rights, in the dignity and worth of the human person and in the equal rights of men and women and have deter-

mined to promote social progress and better standards of life in larger freedom,

Whereas Member States have pledged themselves to achieve, in co-operation with the United Nations, the promotion of universal respect for and observance of human rights and fundamental freedoms,

Whereas a common understanding of these rights and freedoms is of the greatest importance for the full realization of this pledge,

Now, Therefore THE GENERAL ASSEMBLY proclaims THIS UNIVERSAL DECLARATION OF HUMAN RIGHTS as a common standard of achievement for all peoples and all nations, to the end that every individual and every organ of society, keeping this Declaration constantly in mind, shall strive by teaching and education to promote respect for these rights and freedoms and by progressive measures, national and international, to secure their universal and effective recognition and observance, both among the peoples of Member States themselves and among the peoples of territories under their jurisdiction.

Article 1

All human beings are born free and equal in dignity and rights.They are endowed with reason and conscience and should act towards one another in a spirit of brotherhood.

Article 2

Everyone is entitled to all the rights and freedoms set forth in this Declaration, without distinction of any kind, such as race, colour, sex, language, religion, political or other opinion, national or social origin, property, birth or other status. Furthermore, no distinction shall be made on the basis of the political, jurisdictional or international status of the country or territory to which a person belongs, whether it be independent, trust, non-self-governing or under any other limitation of sovereignty.

Article 3

Everyone has the right to life, liberty and security of person.

Article 4

No one shall be held in slavery or servitude; slavery and the slave trade shall be prohibited in all their forms.

Article 5

No one shall be subjected to torture or to cruel, inhuman or degrading treatment or punishment.

Article 6

Everyone has the right to recognition everywhere as a person before the law.

Article 7

All are equal before the law and are entitled without any discrimination to equal protection of the law. All are entitled to equal protection against any discrimination in violation of this Declaration and against any incitement to such discrimination.

Article 8

Everyone has the right to an effective remedy by the competent national tribunals for acts violating the fundamental rights granted him by the constitution or by law.

Article 9

No one shall be subjected to arbitrary arrest, detention or exile.

Article 10

Everyone is entitled in full equality to a fair and public hearing by an independent and impartial tribunal, in the determination of his rights and obligations and of any criminal charge against him.

Article 11

(1) Everyone charged with a penal offence has the right to be presumed innocent until proved guilty according to law in a public trial at which he has had all the guarantees necessary for his defence.
(2) No one shall be held guilty of any penal offence on account of any act or omission which did not constitute a penal offence, under national or international law, at the time when it was committed. Nor shall a heavier penalty be imposed than the one that was applicable at the time the penal offence was committed.

Article 12

No one shall be subjected to arbitrary interference with his privacy, family, home or correspondence, nor to attacks upon his honour and reputation. Everyone has the right to the protection of the law against such interference or attacks.

Article 13

(1) Everyone has the right to freedom of movement and residence within the borders of each state.
(2) Everyone has the right to leave any country, including his own, and to return to his country.

Article 14

(1) Everyone has the right to seek and to enjoy in other countries asylum from persecution.
(2) This right may not be invoked in the case of prosecutions genuinely arising from

non-political crimes or from acts contrary to the purposes and principles of the United Nations.

Article 15

(1) Everyone has the right to a nationality.
(2) No one shall be arbitrarily deprived of his nationality nor denied the right to change his nationality.

Article 16

(1) Men and women of full age, without any limitation due to race, nationality or religion, have the right to marry and to found a family. They are entitled to equal rights as to marriage, during marriage and at its dissolution.
(2) Marriage shall be entered into only with the free and full consent of the intending spouses.
(3) The family is the natural and fundamental group unit of society and is entitled to protection by society and the State.

Article 17

(1) Everyone has the right to own property alone as well as in association with others.
(2) No one shall be arbitrarily deprived of his property.

Article 18

Everyone has the right to freedom of thought, conscience and religion; this right includes freedom to change his religion or belief, and freedom, either alone or in community with others and in public or private, to manifest his religion or belief in teaching, practice, worship and observance.

Article 19

Everyone has the right to freedom of opinion and expression; this right includes freedom to hold opinions without interference and to seek, receive and impart information and ideas through any media and regardless of frontiers.

Article 20

(1) Everyone has the right to freedom of peaceful assembly and association.
(2) No one may be compelled to belong to an association.

Article 21

(1) Everyone has the right to take part in the government of his country, directly or through freely chosen representatives.
(2) Everyone has the right of equal access to public service in his country.
(3) The will of the people shall be the basis of the authority of government; this will shall be expressed in periodic and genuine elections which shall be by universal and equal suffrage and shall be held by secret vote or by equivalent free voting procedures.

Article 22

Everyone, as a member of society, has the right to social security and is entitled to realization, through national effort and international co-operation and in accordance with the organization and resources of each State, of the economic, social and cultural rights indispensable for his dignity and the free development of his personality.

Article 23

(1) Everyone has the right to work, to free choice of employment, to just and favourable conditions of work and to protection against unemployment.
(2) Everyone, without any discrimination, has the right to equal pay for equal work.
(3) Everyone who works has the right to just and favourable remuneration ensuring for himself and his family an existence worthy of human dignity, and supplemented, if necessary, by other means of social protection.

(4) Everyone has the right to form and to join trade unions for the protection of his interests.

Article 24

Everyone has the right to rest and leisure, including reasonable limitation of working hours and periodic holidays with pay.

Article 25

(1) Everyone has the right to a standard of living adequate for the health and well-being of himself and of his family, including food, clothing, housing and medical care and necessary social services, and the right to security in the event of unemployment, sickness, disability, widowhood, old age or other lack of livelihood in circumstances beyond his control.
(2) Motherhood and childhood are entitled to special care and assistance. All children, whether born in or out of wedlock, shall enjoy the same social protection.

Article 26

(1) Everyone has the right to education. Education shall be free, at least in the elementary and fundamental stages. Elementary education shall be compulsory. Technical and professional education shall be made generally available and higher education shall be equally accessible to all on the basis of merit.
(2) Education shall be directed to the full development of the human personality and to the strengthening of respect for human rights and fundamental freedoms. It shall promote understanding, tolerance and friendship among all nations, racial or religious groups, and shall further the activities of the United Nations for the maintenance of peace.

(3) Parents have a prior right to choose the kind of education that shall be given to their children.

Article 27

(1) Everyone has the right freely to participate in the cultural life of the community, to enjoy the arts and to share in scientific advancement and its benefits.
(2) Everyone has the right to the protection of the moral and material interests resulting from any scientific, literary or artistic production of which he is the author.

Article 28

Everyone is entitled to a social and international order in which the rights and freedoms set forth in this Declaration can be fully realized.

Article 29

(1) Everyone has duties to the community in which alone the free and full development of his personality is possible.
(2) In the exercise of his rights and freedoms, everyone shall be subject only to such limitations as are determined by law solely for the purpose of securing due recognition and respect for the rights and freedoms of others and of meeting the just requirements of morality, public order and the general welfare in a democratic society.
(3) These rights and freedoms may in no case be exercised contrary to the purposes and principles of the United Nations.

Article 30

Nothing in this Declaration may be interpreted as implying for any State, group or person any right to engage in any activity or to perform any act aimed at the destruction of any of the rights and freedoms set forth herein.

Appendix 3
Patient's Charter

Extract from Patient's Charter used by Dundee Teaching Hospitals Trust.

We believe you have a right –

- to be treated as an individual, with courtesy, and respect for your dignity, privacy, beliefs and culture
- to equal access, as promptly as possible, to proper and efficient attention from appropriately trained staff
- to be introduced to those providing you with care and to be provided with clear and understandable information about available services
- to be informed about, and involved in, all aspects of your condition and proposed care, with access to your health records with safeguards

- to be offered choices wherever possible in relation to your treatment
- to decide whether or not to participate in medical teaching and research
- to be guaranteed confidentiality of information relating to your care
- to be accommodated in safe, clean and comfortable surroundings
- to be provided with continuity of care as required within and between different health services, including those in the community
- to receive practical help, information and advice about healthier living for you and your family, in relation to nutrition, exercise, smoking and alcohol.

Appendix 4
The Nuremberg code

The great weight of the evidence before us is to the effect that certain types of medical experiments on human beings, when kept within reasonably well-defined bounds, conform to the ethics of the medical profession generally. The protagonists of the practice of human experimentation justify their views on the basis that such experiments yield results for the good of society that are unprocurable by other methods or means of study. All agree, however, that certain basic principles must be observed in order to satisfy moral, ethical and legal concepts:

1. The voluntary consent of the human subject is absolutely essential. This means that the person involved should have legal capacity to give consent; should be so situated as to be able to exercise free power of choice, without the intervention of any element of force, fraud, deceit, duress, over-reaching, or other ulterior form of constraint or coercion; and should have sufficient knowledge and comprehension of the elements of the subject matter involved as to enable him to make an understanding and enlightened decision. This latter element requires that before the acceptance of an affirmative decision by the experimental subject there should be made known to him the nature, duration, and purpose of the experiment; the method and means by which it is to be conducted; all inconveniences and hazards reasonably to be expected; and the effects upon his health or person which may possibly come from his participation in the experiment.
2. The duty and responsibility for ascertaining the quality of the consent rests upon each individual who initiates, directs or engages in the experiment. It is a personal duty and responsibility which may not be delegated to another with impunity.
3. The experiment should be such as to yield fruitful results for the good of society, unprocurable by other methods or means of study, and not random and unnecessary in nature.
4. The experiment should be so designed and based on the results of animal experimentation and a knowledge of the natural history of the disease or other problem under study that the anticipated results will justify the performance of the experiment.
5. The experiment should be so conducted as to avoid all unnecessary physical and mental suffering and injury.
6. No experiment should be conducted where there is an *a priori* reason to believe that death or disabling injury will occur; except, perhaps, in those experiments where the experimental physicians also serve as subjects.
7. The degree of risk to be taken should never exceed that determined by the humanitarian importance of the problem to be solved by the experiment.
8. Proper preparations should be made and adequate facilities provided to protect the experimental subject against even remote possibilities of injury, disability, or death.
9. The experiment should be conducted only by scientifically qualified persons. The highest degree of skill and care should be required through all stages of the experiment of those who conduct or engage in the experiment.

10. During the course of the experiment the human subject should be at liberty to bring the experiment to an end if he has reached the physical or mental state where continuation of the experiment seems to him to be impossible. During the course of the experiment the scientist in charge must be prepared to terminate the experiment at any stage, if he has probably cause to believe, in the exercise of the good faith, superior skill and careful judgment required of him that a continuation of the experiment is likely to result in injury, disability, or death to the experimental subject.

Taken from: Trials of War Criminals before the Nuremberg Military Tribunals under Control Council Law No. 10. Nuremberg, October 1946–April 1949. Washington DC: US GPO, 1949–1953.

Appendix 5

Phases (or 'stages') of clinical trials

Phase one

- Aim to confirm safety at dosage levels anticipated for patients
- Pharmacokinetics and pharmacodynamics are studied intensively and 'surrogate' evidence of activity is sought
- Healthy volunteers frequently studied, except where toxicity expected
- Placebo comparison often present
- Usually numbers of participants small (in order of tens)

Phase two

- Aim to demonstrate efficacy of new agent in disease for which it is intended
- Necessarily real patients as participants
- Participation by appropriate patients requested by researcher
- Participants are consenting recruits rather than volunteers
- Comparison with placebo or with established agent always features
- Usually larger numbers of patients involved (in order of hundreds)

Phase three

- Aim is to show that new agent is superior to existing (in various ways)
- Comparison made between new agent, existing therapy and where feasible, placebo
- Usually 'double blinded', i.e. neither doctors nor patients know what on
- Potential recruits are informed of trial design before giving their consent
- Very large numbers of participants required (in order of thousands)
- Results used as basis for request for licensing by regulatory bodies

Phase four

- Conducted **after** agent is licensed and marketed
- Aim to determine longer term efficacy and safety
- Placebo use not usual
- Often used to refine dose regimes for optimal efficacy
- Can be route to identifying why some patients do not respond
- Numbers of participants variable

Appendix 6

World Medical Association Declaration of Helsinki

Ethical principles for medical research involving human subjects

Adopted by the 18th WMA General Assembly Helsinki, Finland, June 1964 and amended by the 29th WMA General Assembly, Tokyo, Japan, October 1975 35th WMA General Assembly, Venice, Italy, October 1983 41st WMA General Assembly, Hong Kong, September 1989 48th WMA General Assembly, Somerset West, Republic of South Africa, October 1996 and the 52nd WMA General Assembly, Edinburgh, Scotland, October 2000

A. Introduction

1. The World Medical Association has developed the Declaration of Helsinki as a statement of ethical principles to provide guidance to physicians and other participants in medical research involving human subjects. Medical research involving human subjects includes research on identifiable human material or identifiable data.
2. It is the duty of the physician to promote and safeguard the health of the people. The physician's knowledge and conscience are dedicated to the fulfillment of this duty.
3. The Declaration of Geneva of the World Medical Association binds the physician with the words, 'The health of my patient will be my first consideration,' and the International Code of Medical Ethics declares that, 'A physician shall act only in the patient's interest when providing medical care which might have the effect of weakening the physical and mental condition of the patient.'

4. Medical progress is based on research which ultimately must rest in part on experimentation involving human subjects.
5. In medical research on human subjects, considerations related to the well-being of the human subject should take precedence over the interests of science and society.
6. The primary purpose of medical research involving human subjects is to improve prophylactic, diagnostic and therapeutic procedures and the understanding of the aetiology and pathogenesis of disease. Even the best proven prophylactic, diagnostic, and therapeutic methods must continuously be challenged through research for their effectiveness, efficiency, accessibility and quality.
7. In current medical practice and in medical research, most prophylactic, diagnostic and therapeutic procedures involve risks and burdens.
8. Medical research is subject to ethical standards that promote respect for all human beings and protect their health and rights. Some research populations are vulnerable and need special protection. The particular needs of the economically and medically disadvantaged must be recognized. Special attention is also required for those who cannot give or refuse consent for themselves, for those who may be subject to giving consent under duress, for those

who will not benefit personally from the research and for those for whom the research is combined with care.

9. Research Investigators should be aware of the ethical, legal and regulatory requirements for research on human subjects in their own countries as well as applicable international requirements. No national ethical, legal or regulatory requirement should be allowed to reduce or eliminate any of the protections for human subjects set forth in this Declaration.

B. Basic principles for all medical research

10. It is the duty of the physician in medical research to protect the life, health, privacy, and dignity of the human subject.

11. Medical research involving human subjects must conform to generally accepted scientific principles, be based on a thorough knowledge of the scientific literature, other relevant sources of information, and on adequate laboratory and, where appropriate, animal experimentation.

12. Appropriate caution must be exercised in the conduct of research which may affect the environment, and the welfare of animals used for research must be respected.

13. The design and performance of each experimental procedure involving human subjects should be clearly formulated in an experimental protocol. This protocol should be submitted for consideration, comment, guidance, and where appropriate, approval to a specially appointed ethical review committee, which must be independent of the investigator, the sponsor or any other kind of undue influence. This independent committee should be in conformity with the laws and regulations of the country in which the research experiment is performed. The committee has the right to monitor ongoing trials. The researcher has the obligation to provide monitoring information to the committee,

especially any serious adverse events. The researcher should also submit to the committee, for review, information regarding funding, sponsors, institutional affiliations, other potential conflicts of interest and incentives for subjects.

14. The research protocol should always contain a statement of the ethical considerations involved and should indicate that there is compliance with the principles enunciated in this Declaration.

15. Medical research involving human subjects should be conducted only by scientifically qualified persons and under the supervision of a clinically competent medical person. The responsibility for the human subject must always rest with a medically qualified person and never rest on the subject of the research, even though the subject has given consent.

16. Every medical research project involving human subjects should be preceded by careful assessment of predictable risks and burdens in comparison with foreseeable benefits to the subject or to others. This does not preclude the participation of healthy volunteers in medical research. The design of all studies should be publicly available.

17. Physicians should abstain from engaging in research projects involving human subjects unless they are confident that the risks involved have been adequately assessed and can be satisfactorily managed. Physicians should cease any investigation if the risks are found to outweigh the potential benefits or if there is conclusive proof of positive and beneficial results.

18. Medical research involving human subjects should only be conducted if the importance of the objective outweighs the inherent risks and burdens to the subject. This is especially important when the human subjects are healthy volunteers.

19. Medical research is only justified if there is a reasonable likelihood that the populations in which the research is carried out

stand to benefit from the results of the research.

20. The subjects must be volunteers and informed participants in the research project.

21. The right of research subjects to safeguard their integrity must always be respected. Every precaution should be taken to respect the privacy of the subject, the confidentiality of the patient's information and to minimize the impact of the study on the subject's physical and mental integrity and on the personality of the subject.

22. In any research on human beings, each potential subject must be adequately informed of the aims, methods, sources of funding, any possible conflicts of interest, institutional affiliations of the researcher, the anticipated benefits and potential risks of the study and the discomfort it may entail. The subject should be informed of the right to abstain from participation in the study or to withdraw consent to participate at any time without reprisal. After ensuring that the subject has understood the information, the physician should then obtain the subject's freely-given informed consent, preferably in writing. If the consent cannot be obtained in writing, the non-written consent must be formally documented and witnessed.

23. When obtaining informed consent for the research project the physician should be particularly cautious if the subject is in a dependent relationship with the physician or may consent under duress. In that case the informed consent should be obtained by a well-informed physician who is not engaged in the investigation and who is completely independent of this relationship.

24. For a research subject who is legally incompetent, physically or mentally incapable of giving consent or is a legally incompetent minor, the investigator must obtain informed consent from the legally authorized representative in accordance with applicable law. These groups should not be included in research unless the research is necessary to promote the health of the population represented and this research cannot instead be performed on legally competent persons.

25. When a subject deemed legally incompetent, such as a minor child, is able to give assent to decisions about participation in research, the investigator must obtain that assent in addition to the consent of the legally authorized representative.

26. Research on individuals from whom it is not possible to obtain consent, including proxy or advance consent, should be done only if the physical/mental condition that prevents obtaining informed consent is a necessary characteristic of the research population. The specific reasons for involving research subjects with a condition that renders them unable to give informed consent should be stated in the experimental protocol for consideration and approval of the review committee. The protocol should state that consent to remain in the research should be obtained as soon as possible from the individual or a legally authorized surrogate.

27. Both authors and publishers have ethical obligations. In publication of the results of research, the investigators are obliged to preserve the accuracy of the results. Negative as well as positive results should be published or otherwise publicly available. Sources of funding, institutional affiliations and any possible conflicts of interest should be declared in the publication. Reports of experimentation not in accordance with the principles laid down in this Declaration should not be accepted for publication.

C. Additional principles for medical research combined with medical care

28. The physician may combine medical research with medical care, only to the extent that the research is justified by its potential prophylactic, diagnostic or

therapeutic value. When medical research is combined with medical care, additional standards apply to protect the patients who are research subjects.

29. The benefits, risks, burdens and effectiveness of a new method should be tested against those of the best current prophylactic, diagnostic, and therapeutic methods. This does not exclude the use of placebo, or no treatment, in studies where no proven prophylactic, diagnostic or therapeutic method exists.

30. At the conclusion of the study, every patient entered into the study should be assured of access to the best proven prophylactic, diagnostic and therapeutic methods identified by the study.

31. The physician should fully inform the patient which aspects of the care are related to the research. The refusal of a patient to participate in a study must never interfere with the patient-physician relationship.

32. In the treatment of a patient, where proven prophylactic, diagnostic and therapeutic methods do not exist or have been ineffective, the physician, with informed consent from the patient, must be free to use unproven or new prophylactic, diagnostic and therapeutic measures, if in the physician's judgement it offers hope of saving life, re-establishing health or alleviating suffering. Where possible, these measures should be made the object of research, designed to evaluate their safety and efficacy. In all cases, new information should be recorded and, where appropriate, published. The other relevant guidelines of this Declaration should be followed.

Index

Page numbers in *italic* refer to boxed case study material.